TIME FOR HEALING

TIME FOR HEALING

**Integrating Traditional Therapies
with Scientific Medical Practice**

Carl Becker

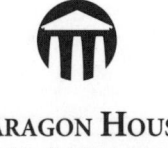

PARAGON HOUSE
St. Paul, Minnesota

Published in the United States of America by

Paragon House Publishers
2700 University Avenue West
St. Paul, Minnesota 55114

Copyright © 2002 by

All rights reserved. Except for use in reviews, no part of this book may be reproduced, stored in a retrieval system, or transmitted in any form or by any means, electronic, mechanical or otherwise, without the prior written consent of the publisher. Copyrights on chapters noted at the end of each chapter.

An ICUS Book

The International Conference on the Unity of the Sciences (ICUS), a project of the International Cultural Foundation, convenes distinguished scientists and scholars to pursue theoretical and practical concerns through an interdisciplinary approach.

Library of Congress Cataloging-in-Publication Data

Becker, Carl B., 1951-
  Time for healing : integrating traditional therapies with scientific medical practice / Carl Becker.—1st ed.
    p. cm.
  Includes bibliographical references and index.
  ISBN 1-55778-820-0 (pbk. : alk. paper)
  1. Alternative medicine. I. Title.
  R733 .B43 2002
  615.5--dc21
                              2002011916

10 9 8 7 6 5 4 3 2 1

For current information about all releases from Paragon House,
visit the web site at http://www.paragonhouse.com

Contents

Introduction

1. Time for Healing: An Introduction to the Problems and Prospects of Integrating Complementary Medicine
   Carl Becker *1*

A "New Age" of Medicine? Educating and Cooperating for a Healthier Public

2. Integrating Science and Nature in a Global Health Care System
   H. Ron Hobbs *13*

3. The Integration of Holistic and Conventional Health Care
   R. Paul Thomlinson *29*

Not Just Skin Deep: Treating Deeper Problems with Different Paradigms

4. Acupuncture in the Modern World
   Daniel Kenner *57*

5. Successful Energetic Treatment of Chronic Depression
   C. Norman Shealy and R. Paul Thomlinson *79*

Not Just Smelling the Flowers: Acquiring Recognition for Aromatherapists

6. Aromatherapy: Healing Aspects of Essential Oils
   Gerry DePaula *99*

7. Holistic Aromatherapy in the United States
   Lizette Pirtle and Sylla Sheppard-Hanger *131*

Not Just an Apple a Day: Researching and Regulating Medicinal Herbs and Plants

8. The Potential of Modern Phytotherapy as a Whole-System Science
   Daniel Kenner *169*

9. Phytotherapy: Challenges for the 21st Century
   Kerry Bone *187*

The Body as a Barometer of the Mind

10. Comprehensive Medicine: Its Philosophy and Methodology
    Katsutaro Nagata. *217*
11. The Changing Faces of Disease and Psycho-Spiritual Healing
    Carl Becker. *247*

1.

Time for Healing

An Introduction to the Problems and Prospects of Integrating Complementary Medicine

Despite the trumpeted advances of biotechnology, the costs and impersonality of modern biomedicine can be troubling. In the wake of awesome advances in scientific medicine, many patients find that doctors don't look at them as friends any more. Not only is the house call a thing of the past. When the patient goes to a modern hospital or HMO, she fills out countless forms, signs informed consent papers, talks to receptionists and nurses, waits for an hour, and then at last has a few minutes with her physician. Her physician looks at the papers that the receptionist handed her, or perhaps at a computer screen where the patient's "data" is already flickering. A nod to the patient, a few strokes on a prescription pad, and the appointment is almost over. If the patient ignores the doctor's glances at her watch and begins to explain what's been troubling her, she's likely to be told "that's not my department," or "get back to me in a couple weeks after taking this prescription."

To complicate things, the prescription is not always effective or without side effects. The patient finds herself paying more for insurance and hospital services than she used to pay her old home doctor, but the pricey medicines leave her more hung-over and upset than the old aspirin, orange juice, and rest that her mother's doctor used to prescribe. Come to think of it, the HMO didn't recommend *rest* at all—didn't even notice the shadowy circles under her eyes or the tired tone in her voice—didn't treat the patient as a person. The patient has been treated much like the car she left in the shop: it will get a lube job and a diagnostic printout. The difference is that the patient has feelings, and those feelings may significantly affect her prognosis and healing outcome, not to mention her future choice of health care providers.

If this is not your doctor or HMO, you can consider yourself fortunate. Happily, a growing number of doctors are receiving training in treating their patients as whole and complex persons—and a growing number of HMOs are beginning to realize that their patient satisfaction will affect their bottom lines in the future. But there still is a long way to go. Facing these circumstances, nearly half the households in America are turning to methods of healing and health-preservation known as "alternative," "complementary," "comprehensive," "traditional," or "holistic." The precise interpretation of these terms varies from practitioner to practitioner; some of the chapters in this book make more precise definitions for their specific contexts and purposes. Let's call them CAM (Complementary Alternative Medicine), for the time being. The important differences between these CAM approaches and the modern Western HMO are that: (1) they put the patient—complete with feelings, hopes, stresses, frustrations, and worldviews—right in the center of their treatment, and (2) they complement the "standard" medical therapy with dietary supplements, aromas, acupuncture, and changes of attitude. By looking at the person as an integral whole, and considering the person's whole life picture, these approaches enable healing not only of obvious superficial medical problems, but sometimes of deeper lifestyle problems that in fact threaten the patient's future health. By using dietary supplements, aromas, acupuncture, and the like, patients reduce their stress, their susceptibility to fatigue and disease, even their pain and side effects from other prescription drugs.

CAM is no panacea; it cannot replace most standard medical practices. Patients should consult their primary care physicians about the CAM practices they are using or contemplating—especially herbs which might interact with other prescriptions. This has been difficult in the past. Traditionally-trained MDs have tended to disparage alternative treatments and practitioners even without solid evidence or sound reasons to do so. On their part, alternative practitioners have sometimes claimed more than they could reasonably deliver, and other times counterattacked the medical profession for their closed-mindedness.

Today, CAM is changing—from an unrecognized "underground" movement of home remedies, traditional wisdom, and common knowledge—into an increasingly recognized and scientifically supported body of medical practices. CAM practices are designed to complement, not conflict with, most standard medical practices. They tend to have few side effects, and to be comparatively inexpensive—especially as a growing number of insurance companies provide policies that cover patients' choice of CAM.

There is already a substantial literature on CAM in professional journals. This book brings together experts on CAM—especially of aromatherapy, phytotherapy, and skin stimulation like acupuncture and TENS. These authorities advance the discussion of CAM in two ways largely lacking in the current literature. In addition to carefully documenting the effectiveness of CAM techniques, each authority points out important but little-known breakthroughs in their specialized fields, and acknowledges the limits and cautions that should be observed in each area. Secondly, they all are concerned to address the important policy issues of education, certification, public awareness, and participation of governments and HMOs in providing safer and more cost-effective health-care—the indispensable next steps before CAM can take its place alongside other medical methods. Their goal is not to advertise specific methods, much less to criticise standard Western medicine. Rather, they propose ways that health-providing professionals can cooperate to give patients more humane, effective, and economical care that patients themselves desire.

While Europe and China have been more forward in recognizing a range of healing therapies, only in the past few years have America, Japan, and Australia (the areas represented by our authors) seen movements toward integrating complementary therapies and standard western biomedicine in the same HMOs or health care packages. This is an exciting prospect with many benefits for health economics as well as health maintenance, but it is seldom a painless process, as Thomlinson and others report.

This book is organized into five sections of two chapters each. In each section, one authority provides historical background and emphasizes specific scientific evidence about the effectiveness and safety cautions of the techniques discussed, while the other looks at policy implications for the integration of such techniques into mainstream health care.

In "A 'New Age' of Medicine?", Drs. Hobbs and Thomlinson address ways that the larger traditions of naturopathy and holistic health care are beginning to assume their place alongside of standard western biomedicine.

Our lead-off writer, Dr. H. Ron Hobbs, now at Bastyr University, has had extensive experience in teaching naturotherapy and designing holistic medical programs at universities including Bridgeport, Antioch, and Yale. In his chapter on integrated health care, Dr. Hobbs first surveys the ideas of holism and the history of naturopathy in the United States, showing their compatibility with as well as differences from standard western biomedicine. Then he reports the development of standards and accreditation programs for modern naturopathy education programs in American universities, and notes the increasing acceptability of holistic and naturopathic methods to insurance companies as well.

In his chapter on "Restraining Forces, Impelling Forces, and Lessons Learned," Dr. R. Paul Thomlinson presents a survey of the state of CAM in today's world of health care. He scrupulously analyzes the forces militating for and against the expansion of CAM and its potentials for integration with modern medical health care systems. Echoing other authors' emphasis on treating the whole patient in context, Thomlinson is boldly optimistic about the cost-effectiveness as well as the healing potentials of CAM in cooperation with health care systems. In particular, the detailed lessons he reports, not only from NIH studies, but also from the Hulston Cancer Center at Cox Health Systems, will be of value to planners as well as patients contemplating more balanced and integrated care packages.

"Not Just Skin Deep" introduces Eastern and Western alternatives for relieving pain and depression. The ancient Sino-Japanese practice of acupuncture is complemented by and contrasted with newer techniques of TENS (applying minuscule microscopic electrical currents to the skin). Both are shown to be very useful adjunct therapies for the reduction of pain and depression, exceeding the effectiveness of many more common treatments.

Dr. Daniel Kenner is a California-licensed acupuncturist who has devoted many years to studying acupuncture in Japan and phytotherapy in France, and has taught alternative healing methodologies at a number of universities. (His major book to date is on phytotherapy.) Dr. Kenner begins his chapter on acupuncture with a sweeping but accessible overview of its development in the context of Chinese and Japanese history. He contrasts four different models of acupuncture, showing their applicability for analgesia, for tension and pain relief, and for specific symptom relief. Throughout, his presentation helps the reader understand the ways in which oriental diagnoses evaluate patients very differently than does Western medicine. He cites evidence that acupuncture can be effective against internal complaints ranging from gallstones to inflammation.

Dr. C. Norman Shealy is world-renowned for his medical anthropological studies including psychic healing in the Philippines, and measuring brain and body parameters of psychic healing in the West. More significantly, over the past 30 years, he has worked to bring comprehensive and complementary healing techniques to his patients at the Shealy Wellness Center. In this paper, Shealy and Thomlinson introduce their extensive experience relieving pain with a very low output TENS (transcutaneous electrical nerve stimulator) device. (TENS has no relation to and should *not* be confused with electric shock treatments.) They report remarkably high success rates, based on serotonin measurement as well as patient satisfaction. But they also caution that many more highly-powered TENS devices are less effective, and that all such equipment should be used with professional supervision. The prospects for relieving chronic pain and chronic depression with a portable and inexpensive headset are intriguing indeed.

"Not Just Smelling the Flowers" takes a serious look at the medical applications of essential oils extracted from flowers and herbs. While aromatherapy has recently become very popular in Asia and America, the past decade or two has seen remarkable advances in our understanding of the effects of essential oils—not merely for perfumery, but for clinical and health-maintenance purposes.

Against the popular image that aromatherapy and essential oils are mere cosmetic or aesthetic aids, Dr. Gerry DePaula gives an impressive review of scientific literature. She categorizes essential oil research into anti-microbial (including anti-bacterial and anti-fungal) effects, showing promise for food preservation as well as for human infections; anti-inflammatory effects, reducing a variety of pain and swelling in animals as well as humans; and metabolic effects, proposing exciting implications for diabetes, obesity, and possibly even preventing hardened arteries. She then gives an important overview of standards for oil production and therapist education, that begins to dovetail with the following chapter by Pirtle and Sheppard-Hanger.

Lizette Pirtle and Sylla Sheppard-Hanger are professional aromatherapists who have been central in the advancement of America's National Association for Holistic Aromatherapy (NAHA). Compared to DePaula's purely biochemical approach, Pirtle and Sheppard-Hanger include holistic "psycho-spiritual" aspects of aromatherapy which are qualitative and therefore more difficult to measure. At the same time, they emphasize the challenges of safety, methods of application, and measurement of therapeutic effectiveness. Then they introduce the roles and activities of NAHA in developing standards for aromatherapy education, certification, and product approval. They conclude with important observations on the economic and even environmental ramifications of harvesting wild herbs for therapeutic uses. Coupled with the scientific literature reported by Dr. DePaula, Pirtle and Sheppard-Hanger give a balanced picture of the progress being made—and yet to be made—in this field of growing popularity.

"Not Just An Apple a Day" recognizes that much of our knowledge of pharmaceuticals and drugs in fact originated in our ancestors' collective wisdom about the uses of plants and plant extracts to care for their health. The tremendous market for dietary supplements and herbal remedies has led governments and insurance companies in many developed nations to contemplate regulating as well as researching their uses. This poses both promises and dangers, as our authors explain.

Dr. Kenner's chapter on phytotherapy argues that it can be seen as a "Whole System": a world-view by which to understand patients and wellness, not merely an add-on technique to be subsumed within present biochemical medicine. Kenner illustrates that the same physical manifestations can be interpreted in entirely different ways by disparate cultural paradigms or medical "nosologies." Moving from one paradigm to another renders certain questions that were askable and answerable in the first paradigm unaskable and unanswerable in the second. Kenner's vision covers not only America, but spans European and Asian paradigms and policies as well. He recognizes the dangers of considering herbs merely as the sum of their parts, and of looking for single "active ingredients" within the complex makeup of natural herbs. He makes many important observations about quality standards, and concludes with a persuasive analysis of the cost-effectiveness of phytotherapy.

Phytotherapist Kerry Bone is a well-identified author and a leader of the National Herbalists Association of Australia. He has consented to our inclusion of this edition of his highly-lauded article that originally appeared in the *Townsend Letter for Doctors and Patients*. Outlining numerous challenges to the field of phytotherapy, he gives specific examples of the dangers in each area, and of specific ways that these challenges or dangers may be met. He cites fascinating cases in which, for example, the knowledge of traditional Inca priest-healers has presaged the scientific experiments that distinguished importantly different chemotypes of the same herb. He illustrates the significant contrasts between *in vivo* and *in vitro* studies, and their implications for phytotherapy and regulatory policies. He notes the distortions common in media depictions of herbal therapy, and the folly of overregulation as well as of underregulation by government agencies. In discussing herbal quality, for example, Bone contrasts the quality required for therapeutic chamomile with that required for herbal chamomile, and continues his analogy with wine to discuss the important use of plant products as "preventive" medicine. Like Pirtle and Sheppard-Hanger, Bone also stresses the importance of environmentally sustainable choices and harvesting techniques.

"The Body as a Barometer of the Mind"

In each of the previous sections, the authors advocate not merely supplementing present techniques of diagnosis and treatment, but more importantly a holistic view of patients and their human relationships, in the processes of understanding health and healing disease. This section takes this theory one step further, by directly discussing the psycho-social and psycho-spiritual effects of patients' thinking upon their health and lifestyles. These presentations stress the importance of comprehensive medicine in dealing with the patients' pains and fears, as well as with the more obvious signs of disease itself.

Dr. Katsutaro Nagata is a leading advocate of integrating Eastern, Western, and psychotherapeutic medicine in Japan.

Director of both Japan's Chronic Pain Association and the Japan Society for the Study of Logotherapy, he has personally struggled with and overcome potentially fatal conditions. He recommends a blend of Western diagnostic techniques, Eastern herbal remedies, and psychotherapy that bridges the two and focuses on the *meaning* of the patient's life and health. Drawing upon the psychological techniques of Michael Balint and Viktor Frankl, among others, Dr. Nagata shows that medical interviews can link as well as transcend traditional medical practices. Nagata's discussion of unmanifest diseases—whether he calls them functional or organic—is of particular interest and importance, because he introduces *specific diagnostic methods* for medically testing the patients' levels of health, resistance, and deterioration, using not only interviews and oriental face-color methods but also chemical urinalysis. This is a very exciting development in enabling early detection and treatment of potential problems that have hitherto gone unrecognized or unheeded by patients as well as by physicians.

In the final chapter, I introduce studies of medical anthropology and of healing religions to identify some of the psycho-social and psycho-spiritual variables that affect health and wellness. From Dr. Hobbs' identification of health with holiness, we come full circle to recognize how important mental attitude is to healing and health maintenance.

This book is the product of the dialogue and cooperation of its several authors, who came together at the 22nd ICUS (International Conference on the Unity of the Sciences) Conference, in Seoul, Korea. The authors join in expressing their thanks to ICUS and its Executive Director Greg Breland for making this project possible, and to Gordon Anderson of Paragon House, for helping us see this project through to this published form.

A "New Age" of Medicine?

Educating and Cooperating for a Healthier Public

2.

Integrating Science and Nature in a Global Health Care System

The Role for Modern Naturopathic Medicine

H. Ron Hobbs, N.D.
Bastyr University School of Naturopathic Medicine

Healing

I am not a mechanism, an assembly of various sections. And it is not because the mechanism is working wrongly, that I am ill. I am ill because of the wounds to the soul, to the deep emotional self, and the wounds to the soul take a long, long time; only time can help; and patience, and certain difficult repentance; long, difficult repentance, realization of life's mistake, and the freeing of one's self from the endless repetition of the mistake which mankind at large has chosen to sanctify.

—D. H. Lawrence

On Definitions of Holism and Integrative Medicine

We owe the modern use of the term "holism" to a man who himself integrated African and European, scientist and statesman, warrior and peacemaker. General Jan Christian Smuts was the Prime Minister of South Africa who released Ghandi from a South African jail and later was central to the formation of the United Nations. Smuts was also an Oxford-trained professional biologist, who coined the term "holism" in 1926 to describe nature's tendency to produce wholes (i.e. bodies or organisms) from the ordered grouping of unitary structures. In his famous book, *Holism and Evolution,* Smuts claims that the "whole making, holistic tendency, or Holism, operating in and through particular wholes, is seen at all stages of existence."[1] Smuts' concept of biological holism was analogous to what philosophers had called "organicism" or "vitalism."

Smuts derived his term from the Greek word "holos," meaning "whole." The similarity of these words suggests that they are cognates in Indo-European languages. The English word "whole" is derived from the Old English word "hal" (as in "hale and hearty"), parent of two other modern words: "health" and "holy." For Anglo-Saxons, and possibly for Indo-Europeans in general, the state of being whole, healthy, and holy was so indivisible that it could be described by a single word. Obviously, in modern times we have come to discriminate aspects of this greater wholeness, most notably to distinguish physical and spiritual aspects of health. The concept of holistic health is, in part, an attempt to return to the original integrity of the concept "hal."

This bit of word play points to an ancient linguistic and philosophical difficulty central to the current dialogue and debate concerning holistic or alternative medicine. Wholes are notoriously difficult to put into words. As Lao Tzu begins the *Tao te Ching,* "The Tao that can spoken is not the true Tao." The power to make distinctions in language is indeed useful; however, these distinctions tend to blind us to the reality of the whole. This dialectic can be seen in Smuts' own proposal that "Instead of the animistic, or the mechanistic, or the mathematical universe, we see the genetic, organic, holistic universe."[2] In our culture, where mechanistic perspectives are so prevalent and persuasive, appending the modifier "holistic" to medicine is part of the attempt to transform the institution of organized medicine that has been criticized for ignoring important aspects of the wholeness of human beings. However, if we are to truly understand the import of holistic medicine, we must see it as contributing to a greater whole, the entirety of human health care.

Integrating Science and Nature in a Global Health Care System

There remains a further difficulty. Smuts coined the words holism and holistic to stress an important observation about nature. That observation, like the rose, would be as valid by any other name. However, like many other words, the word holistic has been used to describe things unrelated to its original meaning—sometimes even to focus on particular practices rather than remembering the whole! As Christiane Northrup, past president of the American Holistic Medical Association (AHMA), has pointed out, we all know "so-called 'holistic' practitioners who treated everything as though it were a nutritional deficiency, simply because nutrition was their specialty—and still others, trained in psychology, who treated every problem as if it were emotionally based. Clearly, the concept 'holistic' was much used and little understood."[3]

By the 1960s, the term "holism" was being applied to an integrative movement in nutrition, and also used to describe Gestalt psychology. According to the Oxford English Dictionary, the adjectival form "holistic" was first used to describe a type of medicine by Hoffman et al. in their 1960 *Psychosomatics* article.[4] In 1978, the AHMA was founded to bring together licensed medical doctors (MDs) and doctors of osteopathic medicine (DOs) who practiced holistic medicine.[5] Kenneth Pelletier did much to popularize the concept of "holistic medicine" with the publication of his book by the same name in 1979.[6] By the 1980s, "holistic medicine" was being widely described as alternative to mainstream pharmaceutical/allopathic medicine.

What was called "holistic medicine" in the 1980s and 1990s is now known most commonly as "complementary and alternative medicine" (CAM). It is increasingly recognized that many of the principles and practices of holistic medicine have been practiced by cultures around the world since the dawn of history.[7] The World Health Organization designates such principles and practices "traditional medicine."[8] The terms "holistic" and now "complementary and alternative" medicine (CAM), cover a wide variety techniques and practices that include the traditional healing practices of Western Europe and North America. The western alternative medicine movement is part of a resurgence of interest in traditional medical practices around the world.[9]

The task of being holistic, if possible at all, requires not only the courage to enlarge our thinking, but also the humility to recognize that our perspectives are always partial, no matter how large we become. Practically, this means that we must train practitioners not only with more tools, but also with the abilities to assess both the powers and limitations of those tools. No matter how adept they become with their particular tools, these practitioners must collaborate with others in the health care community—not only with patients, but also with their communities and other caregivers. (Early in my career I was often advised, "there is more holism in the team approach to medicine than there is in any single practitioner.")

So perhaps the term "integrative medicine" more accurately describes this desired state in the practice of health care.[10] However, we must guard lest this term also become an overused but little understood concept. It is easy to fall into the trap of thinking that the integrated system in which we work is a universe adequate unto itself.[11] No matter how well "integrated," no medical system is either complete or exhaustive. Practitioners still must respect diversity and differences of opinion among both providers and recipients of health care. Furthermore, real integration will be difficult and will take time. In a sense, the ideal of integrative, or holistic, medicine is like the ideal of "Health for All." Everyone recognizes that we are unlikely to arrive at the ideal state, but the more we struggle to achieve, and the closer we approach the ideal, the more of the world's citizens will have access to health care that truly benefits them.

American Naturopathy as an Example of the Holistic Health Movement

The "holistic health" movement can be viewed as a part of the perennial struggle between two philosophically divergent views of

Western medicine that have contended with each other since at least classical Greek times.¹² One side of this divide is represented by Asclepius, the Greek god of medicine; the other side is represented by his daughter Hygeia, the goddess of health, whose name gives us the word "hygiene," the "science of health and the prevention of disease."¹³ This struggle is well expressed by Rene Dubos in his classic text, *Mirage of Health: Utopias, Progress & Biological Change*:

> The myths of Hygeia and Asclepius symbolize the never-ending oscillation between two different points of view in medicine. For the followers of Hygeia, health is the natural order of things, a positive attribute to which men are entitled if they govern their lives wisely. According to them, the most important function of medicine is to discover and teach the natural laws which will ensure a man a healthy mind in a healthy body.
>
> More skeptical, or wiser in the ways of the world, the followers of Asclepius believe that the chief role of the physician is to treat disease, to restore health by correcting any imperfections caused by the accidents of birth or life.¹⁴

Nineteenth century America witnessed the growth of holistic hygiene movements that provide an interesting contrast to the physiological medical movements progressing in the universities and hospitals of urban Europe. For example, naturopathy is a uniquely American brand of "integrative medicine." It emerged from the nineteenth century integration of European "nature cures" (water treatments, dietetics, fasting and exercise) with American homeopathy and "eclectic medicine" (the scientific applications of native American and European immigrants' herbal medicines). Along with the public health profession, naturopathy represents the core of the nineteenth century hygiene movement that is properly credited with many of the health advances of the twentieth century.¹⁵

During the twentieth century, conventional biomedicine (also known as "allopathic" medicine) attained hegemony over health care delivery, relegating many descendents of the hygiene movement to subsidiary or alternative roles.[16] The holistic health movement since the 1970s represents the latest resurgence of the Hygeian tradition, largely in response to the perceived mechanization and depersonalization of modern biomedicine. Today's holistic health movement recalls a number of nineteenth century "medical sects" such as "homeopathy, herbalism, and naturopathy."[17] American naturopathy, rechristened naturopathic medicine, is experiencing a resurgence that started with the holistic health movement and continues unabated with the accelerating interest in complementary and alternative medicine (CAM). This is in part due to the fact that naturopathic medicine appears to be "pre-adapted to the philosophy and therapeutic techniques of the holistic health movement."[18] No doubt it is also because modern naturopathic physicians are unique in North America because they are trained to integrate a comprehensive array of CAM therapies.[19]

What is a Naturopathic Physician?

The terms *naturopathy* and *naturopathic medicine* were coined in nineteenth century America, but some principles of naturopathic medicine go back thousands of years. A syncretistic system of healing, naturopathy today draws on the healing wisdom of the world's traditional cultures, including Ayurvedic India, Taoist China, and Hippocratic Greece. Naturopathic physicians are general practitioners of medicine trained in a wide variety of natural therapies. The U.S. Department of Labor defines a naturopathic physician as one who "diagnoses, treats, and cares for patients, using a system of practice that bases its treatment of all physiological functions and abnormal conditions on natural laws governing the body, utilizes physiological, psychological and mechanical methods, such as air, water, heat, earth, phytotherapy (treatment by use of plants), electrotherapy, physiotherapy, minor or orificial surgery, mechanotherapy, naturopathic corrections and manipulation, and all natural methods or modalities, together with natural medicines, natural processed foods, and herbs, and natural remedies...."[20] Thus major surgery and the prescription of most drugs are excluded from naturopathic practice.

Naturopathic medicine is a distinct profession of primary health care whose practitioners, while diagnosing diseases conventionally, are more oriented to prevention, education, and promotion of optimal health and wellness, rather than just treatment of disease. The following principles form the foundation of naturopathic medicine, and are continually reexamined in light of current scientific advances.

- *First Do No Harm.* Preferred are the least invasive diagnostic procedures, treatments and medicinal substances with minimal risk of harmful side effects.
- *Prevention.* Physicians assess risk factors, make early interventions, and promote wellness by supporting patients to create healthy lifestyles.
- *The Healing Power of Nature.* Naturopathic medicine recognizes and encourages the inherent, ordered, and intelligent healing process in each individual.
- *Treatment of the whole person.* Physicians address the complex interactions of a patient's physical, emotional, mental, environmental, genetic, social and spiritual aspects.
- *Identification and treatment of the causes of disease.* Rather than merely eliminate symptoms, physicians identify and remove underlying causes of illness.
- *Doctor as Teacher.* The physician educates and develops patient self-responsibility, and the therapeutic potential of the doctor-patient relationship is valued and cultivated.

Naturopathic medicine integrates centuries-old knowledge of traditional, non-toxic therapies with the best of modern medical diagnostic science and standards of care. The scope of practice includes all aspects of family care, from natural childbirth to geriatrics. Available data suggest that naturopathic physicians are consulted by patients who vary widely both in their ages and chief illnesses.[21]

Education and Clinical Training

Since the beginning of naturopathic medicine as a formal discipline in the twentieth century, high educational standards have been the rule. Although naturopathic medical schools have never had the resources of the better-endowed allopathic and osteopathic medical schools, they have nonetheless striven to train naturopaths in the biomedical sciences as well as natural therapeutics.

Dr. Benedict Lust founded the American College of Naturopathy in New York City late in 1902. By 1927, an American Medical Association study listed twelve naturopathic schools.[22] At one time, Pennsylvania boasted five naturopathic colleges. Hahnemann Medical School in Philadelphia, originally a homeopathic medical school and now an allopathic medical school, used to grant doctoral degrees in naturopathy.

The first professional naturopathic medical societies were formed at the turn of the century, and some naturopathic medical conventions in the 1920s attracted more than 10,000 practitioners. There were two dozen naturopathic medical colleges, including the dozen listed by the AMA, and physicians were licensed in a majority of states.[23]

After experiencing a decline in the 1940s and 1950s due to the rising popularity of technological medicine, pharmaceutical drugs, and the hope that drugs could eliminate all disease, naturopathic medicine today is experiencing a renaissance, as a health conscious public turns to alternative treatment modalities. A national professional organization for naturopathic physicians was founded in the early 1980s, the American Association of Naturopathic Physicians, to promote the development of credible, science-based naturopathic medicine.

Naturopathic methods are well supported by scientific research in peer-reviewed journals from disciplines including conventional medicine, European complementary medicine, clinical nutrition, Oriental medicine, phytotherapy (herbal medicine), pharmacognosy, homeopathy, psychology and others. A two-volume *Textbook of Natural Medicine*, published by Bastyr University, cites over five thousand references in the scientific literature documenting the efficacy of naturopathic therapies. Published research may also be found in *The Journal of Naturopathic Medicine*. Tools like information technology, statistical analyses, and new emphases in clinical outcomes assessment (such as evidence-based medicine) are particularly suited to evaluating the effectiveness of naturopathic treatment protocols, and increasingly are being used in research at naturopathic medical schools and in the offices of practicing physicians.

Modern naturopathic medicine is committed to the integration of the ancient wisdom of healing with the modern science of biomedicine. While this tendency has been present from the beginning of naturopathy, it is best exemplified by the founding of the John Bastyr College of Naturopathic Medicine in 1978 in the city of Seattle, Washington, USA. Now known as Bastyr University, it has become the first true research institute in the naturopathic profession, operating programs in acupuncture, nutrition, and health psychology. In 1994 Bastyr received one of the first research grants from the NIH Office of Alternative Medicine.

Modern naturopathic medical colleges are four-year professional schools with admission requirements comparable to those of conventional medical schools. There are currently five schools in North America qualified to educate naturopathic physicians: Bastyr University School of Naturopathic Medicine, Canadian College of Naturopathic Medicine, National College of Naturopathic Medicine, Southwest College of Naturopathic Medicine, and the University of Bridgeport College of Naturopathic Medicine (UBCNM). UBCNM is the first naturopathic medical school to operate in the eastern half of America in over 50 years and the first founded within a regionally accredited university. Other universities have announced plans to start naturopathic medical programs.

Modern educational standards for naturopathic physicians became official when the Council on Naturopathic Medicine received recognition from the U.S. Department of Education in 1987. These standards involve completion of a pre-medical education followed by a four-year residential curriculum with 4,500–5,000 hours of instruction. Basic medical science and clinical diagnostic skills are taught during the first two years. The core therapeutic curriculum includes instruction in acupuncture, nutritional sciences, counseling, botanical medicine, homeopathy, Oriental medicine, childbirth, physiotherapy, naturopathic manipulation, minor surgery, and other medical procedures. Students undergo extensive supervised clinical training in outpatient naturopathic clinics. One of the challenges of the profession is to create residency positions to strengthen the clinical postgraduate training.

Graduates of approved programs are eligible to take the Naturopathic Physicians Licensing Exam (NPLEX), offered by the North American Board of Naturopathic Examiners. These exam results are currently used for licensing naturopathic physicians by eleven states and one territory: Alaska, Arizona, Connecticut, Hawaii, Maine, Montana, New Hampshire, Oregon, Puerto Rico, Utah, Vermont and Washington. (The District of Columbia registers naturopaths who have licensure elsewhere.) At least two of the five Canadian provinces that license naturopaths (British Columbia and Ontario) also acknowledge the results of the NPLEX.

Recent Trends in America

Traditionally, naturopathic physicians have worked in private office settings. An increasing trend, particularly in western states, is the establishment of associated practices and interdisciplinary clinics that bring together the services of a diverse group of practitioners. Naturopaths refer their patients to other health care professionals, such as MD's, specialists, and chiropractors whenever appropriate.

However, the venues available for practice are changing. In 1994, the Washington State Department of Health designated naturopathic physicians as one category of "general care providers." Naturopaths in Washington State are now eligible to have their medical school loans forgiven if they agree to work in one of the medically under-served areas of the state. More recently a law was passed which mandated that insurers cover all categories of licensed providers, which include naturopathic physicians and acupuncturists. In response to this, several HMOs include card-carrying naturopathic physicians as primary care providers in their networks.

Another exciting development is the creation of integrated settings where naturopathic physicians work together with their allopathic counterparts. In 1996, Seattle/King County Department of Health opened the Natural Health Clinic in an existing community health center in South King County. A team of allopathic doctors, naturopathic doctors, nutritionists and acupuncturist provide therapy to a community that includes citizens who all too often have not had access to competent practitioners of complementary medicine.

In 1998, Cancer Treatment Centers of America, a hospital-based program that had long offered nutritional therapies to its cancer patients, inaugurated a Naturopathic Medical Program in its hospitals. CTCA now employs naturopathic doctors and residents in two of their hospitals.

In 1999, the University of Bridgeport College of Naturopathic Medicine (UBCNM) collaborated with the Yale/Griffin Prevention Research Center in Derby, Connecticut, to open an Integrated Medical Clinic.[24] The Clinic is co-directed by Dr. David Katz (MD) of the Yale University School of Medicine, and Dr. Christine Girard-Couture (ND) of the clinical faculty at UBCNM. All of these developments have been exceedingly popular with the patients who use these facilities.

Today's health care crisis, with its spiraling costs and the rising number of chronic degenerative diseases too often unresponsive to current treatments, has stimulated the renewal of naturopathic medicine and traditionally-based alternative healing modalities. More and more people are choosing natural medicine for primary care or in conjunction with conventional treatment. Naturopathic medicine offers many documented short and long-term cost containment benefits and, with its emphasis on causation, prevention, health promotion and lifestyle changes, will play an important role in shifting our health care system from a disease to a wellness orientation.

A Global Perspective

The movement to integrate traditional and modern hygiene and medicine in order to provide appropriate health is not limited to the naturopathic profession, much less to the developed world. In a curious example of synchronicity, in the same year that Bastyr University was founded, the World Health Organization met on the other side of the globe in Alma Ata, Kazakhstan, to formulate the goal of "Health for All." This audacious goal mandated that health officials work toward providing primary health care for all the citizens of this planet. The WHO recognized that one important way to accomplish this would be to foster cooperation and mutual respect between traditional and modern practitioners. Only a year earlier, the Thirtieth World Health Assembly had adopted a resolution that traditional medicine should promote and integrate with modern Western medicine.[25]

Recently the World Health Organization estimated that probably 80 percent of the world's population has access only to traditional medicine, known to the Western world as "alternative" medicine. From a global perspective, this medicine is hardly alternative. Common sense suggests that the delivery of primary health care to all of the citizens of the world will require the integration of traditional and modern medicine. While most researchers have focused on the examples of traditional Oriental medicine and Ayurvedic medicine, the American experiment with naturopathic medicine really represents the modern development of the traditional medicine of Europe and North America. Its struggles with the difficult concept of integration also provide a roadmap for the integration of traditional medicine that is happening throughout the modern world's "global village." This process is an important part of what might be called the "globalization" of health care at both the local and global levels.

For all of its technical prowess, modern Western medicine has disregarded many traditionally wise and humane ways of looking at hygiene, health, and disease, as well as many techniques that potentially promote health and well-being. Governments as well as private insurance companies are coming to realize that, in order to provide affordable health care, countries and health care systems have to find ways of integrating the principles and practices of traditional heath care, whether they be called holistic, alternative, complementary, or natural medicine.

Notes

1. Smuts, J. C., *Holism and Evolution.* New York: MacMillan, 1926, 1961.

2. Smuts, quoted in *Oxford English Dictionary Online*, "holism."

3. Northrup, C. Foreword. in Altenberg, H.E., *Holistic Medicine: A Meeting of East and West.* Tokyo and NY: Japan Publications, 1992.

4. Hoffman et al. quoted in *Oxford English Dictionary Online*, "psychosomatics."

5. Cf. www.holisticmedicine.org.

6. Pelletier, Kenneth R., *Holistic Medicine.* New York: Delacorte Press, 1979.

7. Akerele, O. "The best of both worlds: bringing traditional medicine up to date." *Social Science and Medicine,* 1987; 24(2):177–181.

8. WHO, *The Promotion and Development of Traditional Medicine.* Tech. Report Serv. 622, 1978.

9. Christie, V. M., "A dialogue between practitioners of alternative (traditional) medicine and modern (Western) medicine in Norway." *Social Science and Medicine,* 1991; 32(5): 549–552.

10. Johnston, C. J. "Integrative Medicine." *Notes from the Edge:* www.creativesystems.org.

11. Johnston, C. M., "Beyond the unity fallacy." Association for Humanistic Psychology *Perspective,* Oct./Nov. 1987, p. 6.

12. Coulter, H. L., *Divided Legacy: A History of the Schism in Medical Thought.* Washington, DC: Wehawken, 1975.

13. Morris, W., ed. *The American Heritage Dictionary of the English Language.* Boston: American Heritage; 1975.

14. Dubos, R.J., *Mirage of Health: Utopias, Progress & Biological Change.* New Brunswick, NJ: Rutgers Univ. Press, 1987 [quoted in the *Bastyr University Catalog,* 1997, p. 22].

15. McKeown, T., *The Role of Medicine: Dream, Mirage, or Nemesis.* London: The Nuffield Provincial Hospitals Trust, 1976, quoted in Banta, D., "What is Health Care?" in Kovner, A. R. (ed), *Health Care Delivery in the United States.* NY: Springer, 1990, pp. 8–30.

16. Starr, P., *The Social Transformation of American Medicine.* New York: Basic Books, 1982.

17. Berliner, H., and Salmon, J. W. "The holistic alternative to scientific medicine: history and analysis." *International Journal of Health Services,* 1980 10: 133–147.

18. Baer, H. A., "The potential rejuvenation of American naturopathy as a consequence of the holistic health movement." *Medical Anthropology,* 1992; 13: 369–383.

19. Boon, H., "Canadian naturopathic practitioners: Holistic and scientific world views." *Soc Sci Med,* 1998 May; 46(9): 1213–25.

20. U.S. Department of Labor, Dictionary of Occupational Titles, Occupations in Medicine and Health.

21. Boon, H., "Canadian naturopathic practitioners: Holistic and scientific world views." *Social Science and Medicine,* 1998 May; 46(9):1213–25.

22. Reed, L., *The Healing Cults.* Chicago: University of Chicago Press; 1932.

23. Baer, H. A., "The potential rejuvenation of American naturopathy as a consequence of the holistic health movement." *Med. Anthro.*, 1992; 13: 369–383.

24. Carvalko, D., "Griffin integrates doctors, naturopaths." *Connecticut Post*, Bridgeport; Dec. 7, 1999: p. A3, also Carvalko, D., "Griffin blends treatment disciplines." *Connecticut Post*, Jan. 13, 2000, p. A4.

25. See sources cited in notes 7–9.

3.

The Integration of Holistic and Conventional Health Care

Restraining Forces, Impelling Forces, and Lessons Learned

R. Paul Thomlinson, Ph.D.
Burrell Behavioral Health

Introduction

Health care innovators and change agents have always been the target of the dominant sector of the establishment, whose goal often appears to be condemnation of any clinical approaches or philosophies that fall outside the prevailing paradigm. Many well-known historical exemplars support this contention; Andreas Vesalius was condemned as a heretic for correcting erroneous sixteenth century anatomical dogma, and the "father of modern surgery," Ambroise Paré, was ridiculed for his precocious use of ligature instead of cauterization during surgical procedures. So it should not be surprising that many attempts to move the biomedical-oriented health care establishment to a more holistic enterprise have been a source of debate, denunciation, and controversy.

Recently, for example, Barrett (2000) condemns alternative medicine proponents for having "…strayed from scientific thought. The factors that motivate them can include delusional thinking, misinterpretation of personal experience, financial considerations, and pleasure derived from notoriety and/or patient adulation." According to Cohen (1998), "In recent years, holistic providers have faced hostile medical boards and organized opposition from segments of the biomedical community," with licensed MDs employing homeopathy, for example, having "had their licenses revoked by state medical boards merely for using" this alternative approach. Additionally, "Licensed nonmedical providers offering nutritional guidance to support the healing process have been prosecuted for practicing medicine without a license, even when authorized by their licensing statutes to provide 'dietary advice.'"

Dossey's (1997) editorial in *Alternative Therapies in Health and Medicine* puts the situation into proper perspective: "The resistance...to CAM [complementary and alternative medicine] conceals a fear that good science may be degraded or contaminated by bad science. Rigid barriers must therefore be erected to keep out the contaminating influences. This may be why [opponents] are so troubled by the integration of CAM with orthodox medicine. To them, integration is a sneaky strategy—the nose of the camel under the tent. To prevent this, orthodox medicine must be segregated from CAM at all costs—CAM apartheid."

If there is to be a significant shift in the biomedical community toward a truly integrated health care system, the two systems must expend time and effort to find ways in which their working together could maximize their patients' well being. As Gruman (1997) notes, "No one in a responsible position is advocating the uncritical acceptance of all alternative medicine practices. Neither is anyone advocating indiscriminate applications of the pharmacological, surgical, and diagnostic interventions that currently constitute standard medical treatment. Rather, the demand is for health care services that work, that reliably reduce morbidity and mortality, that reduce suffering and improve quality of life and functioning." Some of the staunchest critics from the side of conventional biomedicine have made overweening assumptions about the dividing line between the two medical cultures—assumptions that are not shared by many in the holistic health care movement. Dr. C. Norman Shealy, founding president of the American

The Integration of Holistic and Conventional Health Care

Holistic Medical Association, emphasizes that these systems are indeed overlapping and complementary, not contradictory: "Holistic physicians first must practice an acceptable standard of traditional medicine: adequate history, physical examination and appropriate laboratory tests similar to those in any competent physician's practice. The holistically oriented physician, however, in addition to standard diagnostic tests, must look at the patient from the point of view of total distress." (Shealy, 1980).

To more fully understand the possible synergies between conventional and holistic systems of medicine, we should consider the questions of (1) *whether the systems can be integrated*, (2) *risks, barriers and benefits of integration*, and (3) *lessons learned* from past and current integration efforts.

Can Holistic Medicine Be Integrated into the Mainstream?

The question of whether holistic medicine can be integrated into existing conventional systems quickly leads to another question: Do holistic and alternative practitioners in their respective nations have the collective desire, resources, and political will to lay the foundation necessary to achieve this goal? The answer to this question remains unclear at present, but it is instructive to consider what this "foundation" might require. Stated simply, "alternative medicine must develop a collective infrastructure.... Practitioners are now talking about adding to the artistry of their alternative practices the dimension of science. The way to do this in science is to eliminate the bias of the single observer...alternative medicine practitioners must, within their disciplines or professions, undergo a parallel process on an administrative and political level. This means moving away from the model of the individual artist as healer to one that guarantees a standard level of knowledge and competence without, one would hope, losing the element of artistry" (Gruman, 1997).

How might this "parallel process" be accomplished? The following recommendations should be considered elemental in the building of a supportive and durable infrastructure for an integrated holistic system of medicine (Gruman, ibid):

- Whatever the holistic discipline is, the knowledge base that defines it "must become agreed upon, systematized and evaluated." Clinically and scientifically validated knowledge acceptable as a basis for holistic medical practice must be distinguished from unproven theories and folk practices. Of course, this also requires that members of the profession clearly determine and state "what they can do and what they cannot."
- Holistic health care providers must have their own as well as their colleagues' healing work "examined against a set of common assumptions and practices." This important step would require them to "be willing to set in place standards that constitute what they know and do as a profession."
- Furthermore, holistic providers "must be willing to police themselves according to these standards."

By these criteria, holistic medicine is still in the initial stages of building the necessary foundation and networks to shift into the prevailing health care system in many Western countries. Clearly, to do so will require enormous resources, including money, time, energy, patience, and steadfast commitment.

The issue of resources required to build infrastructure leads us to consider an interesting conundrum. Because insurance companies still do not pay for many alternative practices(!), the cost of these services remains relatively low, so they are available to a wide array of consumers who can afford them "out of pocket." Providers offering these services are able to charge less for them precisely because they are not engaging in the costly efforts of building the aforementioned collective infrastructure: governance activities, licensing, certification, examining boards, malpractice coverage, and the like. Moreover, alternative practitioners independent of the mainstream can often reduce administrative costs for referral, contracting, utilization review, and billing activities—all of which are necessary to sustain a "managed care" process.

Ironically, integrating holistic medicine into the mainstream may raise its costs and reduce its attractiveness. Alternative practitioners' investment in the creation of an expensive but ultimately necessary bureaucracy may make their services less affordable to their patients, as the fees for alternative services are inflated to cover the "price of admission" to the medical establishment. This may be too high a price to pay for many of the holistic professions, unless they are convinced that the shift will benefit their patients and their healing art in the long term.

Another major issue for individual practitioners and health care systems considering integration of holistic approaches is liability insurance. Questions of accountability, implied endorsement of approaches or products, and the like, must be thought through and settled before most providers can feel comfortable "playing in this arena." As Weil (1995) has put it, "An atmosphere of distrust has poisoned doctor/patient relationships, so that every patient coming through the door is now seen as a potential plaintiff in a lawsuit. Doctors are more afraid than ever to deviate from conventional standards of practice."

Many other chapters of this book demonstrate that a massive research base supports the use of certain "holistic" treatment modalities. However necessary, perfecting of this research base is insufficient to achieve integration; the same is true of building the professional infrastructure mentioned above. In order to facilitate integration, "it is also necessary to have organizational structures within the health care institutions that have the ability to accommodate the services. The kinds of case management required to use the services of…alternative medicine…effectively are simply not available in most places" (Gruman, 1997). Indeed, even when conventional and alternative practitioners provide their services within the same hospital building or administrative structure, it is imperative that vigorous case management move patients across the continuum of care in appropriate ways.

Risks, Barriers, and Restraining Forces to Integrative Care

As in any widespread attempt to significantly change consciousness and behavior, numerous factors resist integrating holistic approaches into the established medical system. Opposition to change seems a ubiquitous human characteristic; the practice of avoiding risk whenever possible even serves as a type of survival mechanism for established cultures and practices.

Physicians should carefully weigh the serious risks of integration for conventional health care systems. Physicians who integrate holistic approaches into their work have been threatened with deprivation of their professional licenses and loss of hospital privileges, even when there is no evidence of harm or risk to patients from their holistic treatments. This has caused some to turn their backs on the biomedical community at large, to seek funding and publication outlets outside the standard channels, further deepening the rift between the two medical cultures. Additionally, conventional health systems attempting to integrate alternative approaches risk alienating the physician community due to their widespread prejudices that alternative approaches smack of charlatanism or quackery.

Frequently unaware of CAM's massive and growing clinical data base, opponents stridently decry that we lack adequate data to support the benefits claimed by holistic medicine proponents. This is particularly ironic, given the fact that conventional medicine employs many treatments without the rigorous levels of scientific testing demanded by critics of holistic medicine. Referring to conventional biomedicine, Eddy (1993) writes: "the credibility of clinical judgment, whether exercised individually or collectively, has been severely challenged by observations of wide variations in practices, inappropriate care, and practitioner uncertainty.... The presumption that if a treatment is widely used it must have some benefit has been shaken not only by reports that many common treatments have no supporting evidence of effectiveness...but by actual trials that have overturned some common beliefs, such as the value of encainide and flecainide for heart attacks...and steroids for acute optic neuritis."

A more fundamental risk to holistic medicine's core identity is posed by the "price of admission" to the biomedical community. While rigorous research to establish efficacy is widely recognized as a necessary but insufficient condition for acceptance, such a program of research may have unintended or even deleterious effects on holistic medicine. As expressed by Cohen (1998), "Validation satisfactory to the biomedical community may make holistic practice conform to biomedical standards and force holistic therapies into a reductionistic or mechanistic mold (e.g., requiring a prescribed number of acupuncture treatments for a particular condition). Moreover, holistic providers may become just as inclined as biomedical providers to treat patients on an 'assembly line' basis or reduce subtle exchange of *chi* to an insurable event...bringing holistic therapies into a reductionistic, mechanistic model may come at the expense of the focus on wholeness and individuality which makes these therapies distinct."

Another significant barrier to integration, at least in Western medicine, is the overwhelming focus of the health care system on acute care. The allopathic medical developments of this system are truly remarkable. However, a major factor affecting the inclusion of holistic practices is the extent to which health care service providers and policy analysts come to terms with the problems presented by *chronic illness*. To the extent that decision-makers focus on acute care, they may be more resistant to integrative holistic approaches to chronic illness. Medical policy makers ignore chronic illness at their own peril; the mushrooming numbers of the aging and chronically ill call out for attention. Elder care accounts for about 50 percent of most health care systems' patient volume and revenue, so it clearly makes sense to expend more effort on designing programs for chronic illnesses such as arthritis, cancer, or cardiac conditions. This population could especially benefit from specific exercise programs drawn from *tai chi* or yoga, and this population appears very interested in herbal and other "natural" remedies.

The U.S. National Institutes of Health sponsored a meeting of more than two hundred health care leaders and experts with the goals of better defining the domains of alternative health care and recommending research priorities in the area. The landmark report that emerged from this meeting is entitled *Report to the National Institutes of Health on Alternative Medical Systems and Practices in the United States* (1994). In addition to outlining seven major domains of holistic medical practice, it provides a useful perspective on the resistance that alternative practitioners often experience from conventional biomedical physicians. This resistance is framed in terms of a set of "belief barriers" that preclude these physicians from "viewing anything labeled 'alternative' in a positive light." Such barriers include: (a) the notion that there is "one 'true' medical profession," (b) overconfidence and overestimation of the importance of advanced medical technology, (c) feelings of security in maintaining the status quo, and (d) stereotyping that holistic practice "attracts people with 'weak' minds...who easily succumb to the 'sideshow' lures of 'snake oil' salespeople."

These "belief barriers" are related to one of the integration obstacles outlined by Weil (1995), which is that "medical education is frozen in a disease-oriented mode." Weil suggests that "the biomedical model from which medical scientists work stifles movement" in the holistic arena, and "from that model's materialistic perspective, doctors can easily dismiss most of the ideas [of holistic medicine] as unscientific and unworthy of investigation."

The solution to such attitudinal barriers is neither simple nor straightforward, but must include a "radical reform of medical education," involving: (a) "basic instruction in the philosophy of science, with reference to new models based on quantum physics that replace old concepts of Newtonian mechanism and Cartesian dualism," (b) "instruction in the history of medicine with reference to the development of major systems like traditional Chinese medicine, homeopathy, and osteopathy," (c) "emphasis on the healing power of nature and the body's healing system," (d) "emphasis on mind/body interactions, including placebo responses, medical hexing, and psychoneuroimmunology," (e) "instruction in psychology and spirituality in addition to information about the physical body," and (f) "practical experience with the basic techniques of alternative medicine…in addition to the basic techniques of allopathic medicine," among others (Weil, 1995).

There is evidence that some of this "radical reform" may indeed be taking place; in 1996, 60 U.S. medical schools included complementary and alternative medicine subjects in their "existing, required coursework, while another 56 offered it as an elective…only 37 offered no instruction in complementary medicine" (Kuhn, 1999). However, very few nursing schools offer integrated alternative medicine training.

Yet another barrier is the lack of a solid bedrock of clinical cost-effectiveness research. As Gruman (1997) points out, "in an age of accountability and utility, the health professions will only be successful if they can show that they can reliably solve intractable health problems…. To be admitted into conventional care, alternative practitioners have to show not only what they propose is effective, but that it is cost-neutral or cost-beneficial. This information is difficult to come by." While such cost-effectiveness data are hard to obtain, holistic medicine may do well to "borrow a page from the songbook" of behavioral medicine, a discipline that has an ever-deepening pool of so-called "medical cost-offset" research (see Friedman, et al., 1995; and Chiles, Lambert & Hatch, 1999). If holistic approaches are construed as truly complementary to allopathic medicine, rather than as a replacement for the discipline, then the methods of cost-offset research could be readily adapted and applied in domains of holism other than mind-body medicine. But the notion of cost-offset makes no sense in a system that lacks integration of services and accounting; only in a truly integrated system of care does the concept offer significant advantages.

Holistic medicine is often rejected on the grounds that it lacks *well-defined mechanisms of action*, although this is by no means unique to holistic medicine. Conventional medicine also often operates from the perspective of "dustbowl empiricism," in which researchers follow up and verify relationships or mechanisms discovered fortuitously without any overarching theoretical construct. For example, much current practice in psychopharmacology, such as the use of lithium to stabilize the mood swings of patients with bipolar disorder, has come about as a result of "happy accidents" that were later empirically verified. After verification, however, comes the task of more thoroughly mapping out the mechanism(s) responsible for the effects obtained. This is a significant issue for many disciplines under the rubric of holistic medicine. Gruman (1997) has put it this way: "It is not enough merely to know that a given practice works. Understanding how and why it works both strengthens the ability to intervene effectively and contributes more broadly to an understanding of human functioning."

This demand that understanding of medical mechanisms be a criterion for acceptability is a tall order for many holistic practitioners. Yet classic and current psychoneuroimmunology research provides plausible explanations for the well-documented impact of mind-body interventions such as guided imagery, relaxation training, and the like. For example, one of the most notable proponents of holism in health care, Dr. Candace Pert, has done much to advance our understanding of the links between emotions and immune functioning. She summarizes an important set of research findings: "…your brain is extremely well integrated with the rest of your body at a molecular level, so much so that the term *mobile brain* is an apt description of the psychosomatic network through which intelligent information travels from one system to another…the neuropeptides and their receptors are the substrates of emotions, and they are in constant communication with the immune system, the mechanism through which health and disease are created" (Pert, 1997). Although this is just one example specifically related to the role of emotions as mediators of health and illness, the point is that we are making advances in understanding the mechanisms of holistic practice, just as for conventional medical approaches.

Compelling Forces and Benefits of Integration

Public demand for complementary services is clearly a major driver of integration efforts. In a recent survey commissioned by Landmark Healthcare (1998), 45 percent of the respondents were willing to pay higher premiums to have a complementary and alternative medicine (CAM) benefit included in their health insurance, and two-thirds of the respondents indicated that inclusion of such benefits would be important in their selection of a health plan. This demand is undoubtedly fueled by many forces, including: (a) the wellness trend in public consciousness, characterized by dissatisfaction with invasive treatments, and desire for more personal control over and information about health care, (b) frustration with the inadequacies of conventional, allopathic medicine, including its ineffectiveness in preventing or treating chronic conditions, and treatment of symptoms rather than causes, (c) loss of personal, caring relationships with health care providers, in which patients can feel that adequate time and attention is devoted to their questions and concerns.

The American Medical Association's Council on Scientific Affairs (1997) explains it this way: "The failure (real or perceived) of many physicians and medical specialties to understand and practice preventive medicine and to communicate effectively with patients, and conventional medicine's dependence on costly diagnostic and procedural interaction that ignores the human side of medicine, may have helped spur public interest in alternative and unconventional therapy." Astin (1998), in the *Journal of the American Medical Association,* reports that around one-third of survey respondents (30 percent to 34 percent) indicated they used alternative approaches to complement their health care, with only 4 percent utilizing alternative therapies exclusively. Astin's study outlines the attitudinal variables that are significant predictors of the use of alternative medicine. Not surprisingly, these findings include another important dimension: belief in the importance and value of one's inner life and experiences. Further, the study shows that demand for alternative approaches is based on experienced benefits, as evidenced by statements such as "I get relief from my symptoms," "I feel better," or "The treatment works better for my health problem." Astin also reports that the people demanding alternative services tend to have higher incomes and education, a more "holistic approach" to health care, and are likely to agree with the statement, "The treatment promotes health rather than just focusing on illness."

Parents searching for alternatives to invasive, risky, or dangerous-sounding medical treatments for their children represent another drive for integration. Indeed, it seems safe to say that patients are more likely to patronize health care providers who are at least sensitive to the trend of integrating holistic approaches into their care. Providing some level of integrated CAM services shows a consumer responsiveness that may provide an important competitive advantage to doctors and health care systems. Holistic approaches to health care certainly provide market differentiation for many, allowing them to stand out in a sometimes nondescript but fiercely competitive healthcare marketplace.

Holistic approaches have often been pursued as an untapped revenue stream for health care systems that desperately need ways of enhancing their margins. Eisenberg, et al. (1998) reported that consumers spent $27 billion on CAM treatments in 1997 in the

The Integration of Holistic and Conventional Health Care

United States, and current estimates approach $31 billion for 2000 (Emerich, 1999). With those kinds of numbers, it is not surprising that many health care systems have tried their hand at obtaining a "piece of the pie." However, many attempts fail to realize the financial windfalls because "many providers come to integration with an inflated expectation of getting hold of the cash...they built large, expensive facilities that 'simply were not sustainable.' ...Some centers have broken even, fewer have shown profits, and several have taken a bath in red ink" (Thompson, 2000). So even though the promise of economic return can motivate integration, it should not be seen as the primary or sole reason for such efforts. As integrative medicine consultant Linda Bedell Logan puts it, "I ask hospitals, 'Is your intent to increase your income or to change the way healthcare is delivered forever?' If they say it is to pad their bottom line, I tell them they're not going to make it" (cited in Thompson, 2000).

The U.S. federal government also has begun to express active interest in the study and integration of alternative approaches to health care. First, the National Institutes of Health created its Office of Alternative Medicine (OAM) in 1991, with funding beginning at $2 million in the following year. The OAM was upgraded to an NIH Center in 1998 and became the National Center for Complementary and Alternative Medicine (NCCAM), with a 1998 budget of $50 million. One of the major purposes of NCCAM funded research is "to allow validated therapies to be further integrated into conventional medical practice" (Kuhn, 1998). There are now 13 NCCAM funded centers engaged in testing the effectiveness of a variety of holistic health care modalities for conditions including HIV/AIDS, stroke, addictions, asthma, cancer, pain, and women's health.

Another encouraging development for holistic advocates is the March 2000 establishment of The White House Commission on Complementary and Alternative Medicine Policy. This commission provides legislative and administrative guidance for CAM-related education, training, access, and delivery, towards shaping the integration of alternative approaches into conventional medicine. Integration proponents hope this group will make significant strides in systematizing and standardizing the disparate credentialing and payment processes that characterize CAM practice.

Integrated CAM approaches do not require a capital intensive, "bricks and mortar" startup, but are employed to best advantage to enhance existing strategies in health care. That is, holism can provide quality improvement to existing service lines. For example, integrating mind/body medicine approaches can provide enormous benefit to an oncology center. The following case illustrates such an integration, along with some of the benefits of the arrangement:

As advances in medical care have improved cancer survival rates, the importance of psychosocial interventions to help cancer patients deal with diagnosis and treatment has increased dramatically. For the past four years, Burrell Behavioral Health, an affiliate of Cox Health Systems in Springfield, Missouri, has been providing psychosocial and mind/body medicine services to cancer patients through the Hulston Cancer Center. Recognizing that their multidisciplinary team was incomplete, three oncologists sought a psychologist to address the short- and long-term emotional issues that their cancer diagnoses presented their patients.

The clinical psychologist they selected has had remarkable experiences and successes working with both the doctors and their patients. She sees every new chemotherapy patient—in both inpatient and outpatient settings. In her initial visit, she is able to introduce herself and educate the patient about the resources available through the program, such as orientation, information, support groups, an educational class called "Coping with Cancer," individual and family therapy. This initial visit also enables her to assess the patients' support system, and to evaluate their history of depression and anxiety (issues that significantly affect the ability of patients to cope with their new diagnoses). She ensures that the patients also know precisely how to contact her and how to access all of the services she has explained.

In short, patients leave their first visit with the feeling that the psychologist is part of a seamless team with the oncologists and other medical staff at the Hulston Cancer Center. This is a crucial aspect of cancer care, as expressed recently by a breast cancer patient: "The team approach made me feel that I was the center of attention, that everyone's energy was being expended on my well-being and getting me back on track, both physically and emotionally...it's very reassuring to know that you're in competent hands."

Indeed, through this integrated approach to care, Hulston makes available all of the components of effective intervention identified by Fawzy and colleagues (1995) in their famous review of the literature on psychosocial and mind/body approaches to cancer care. The four most frequently described categories are:

Educational techniques, usually to reduce the patients' sense of helplessness and inadequacy due to uncertainty and lack of knowledge. These interventions seek to replace uncertainty with mastery and control, and may cover technical aspects of the disease and treatment as well as information on coping and emotional issues. All five studies reviewed showed *beneficial affective, cognitive, treatment adherence, or knowledge effects*,

Behavioral training, usually to reduce psychological stress, as well as the physical complications and side-effects of cancer treatment. Some of these techniques are progressive muscle relaxation, hypnosis (both self- and therapist-induced), deep breathing, meditation, biofeedback, passive relaxation, guided imagery and visualization. All four studies reviewed demonstrated *convincing effects on anxiety and cortisol levels (stress reduction); several even showed significant effects on immune system parameters* (NK cell activity, mixed lymphocyte responsiveness, etc.) that were directly correlated with the behavioral interventions. The findings argue that this is a very effective intervention.

Individual psychotherapy, the cornerstones of which are support, compassion, and empathy. Studies often fail to report the detailed format of the therapy that they review, but "therapy," "psychotherapy," and "counseling" are the most common terms used. All the studies stress the importance of support and emotional engagement of the patient, regardless of the term used. The 13 studies reviewed were universally supportive of the beneficial physical, emotional, and mortality effects of these individual interventions.

Group interventions may take the form of support groups, coping skills training, or more traditional supportive-expressive group therapy. Typically, problem-oriented and skills-training groups have demonstrated the most effectiveness in outcome studies. Spiegel and colleagues' (1989) classic research on supportive group therapy with metastatic breast cancer patients has shown mean survival lengths for experimental patients to be about twice as long as control patients (36.3 months compared to 18.9 months, respectively).

Often, it is not until late in treatment that patients turn to these important and validated treatment options. But after the initial visit, the patient now has a familiar name and face to call on in the midst of a very unfamiliar experience. It is important to distinguish this approach from the traditional referral model, in which a psychologist sees patients only when they are in crisis. When the treatment team incorporates psychosocial care in their planning, patients more easily understand that a period of psychological adjustment to their new cancer diagnosis is absolutely normal. Significantly, this orientation also increases the likelihood that patients will be comfortable accessing psychosocial care when they need it.

Among the countless benefits of addressing the psychosocial needs of cancer patients and adding a more holistic approach to cancer care are that counseled patients relate better to their physicians and are more likely to adhere to their treatment plans, from taking medications to showing up for appointments. The experience of integrating more holism into cancer care at the Hulston Cancer Center has been overwhelmingly positive for physicians, the mind/body medicine specialist, and patients.

In the future, health systems *not* employing proven alternative strategies in their care may face significant risks. The evidence supporting some CAM practices (e.g., mind-body interventions, supportive group therapy for cancer patients) makes a strong argument for their inclusion in "best practices" guidelines. As the evidence mounts, systems failing to integrate empirically validated alternative methods may face increased risks of litigation for medical negligence.

Lessons Learned from Integration Attempts and Successes

Examples of integration of holism into health care range from capital-intensive approaches developing new building complexes, information systems, health care staffs, and research projects, to the more common approach of inserting holistic approaches into existing service lines. Many health care systems are surprised when they "take inventory" of the array of services they are already providing that fall under the rubric of holistic or CAM approaches. Even the most conservative and conventional of health care systems probably have on their staffs nutritionists with deep interests in herbal medicine and other dietary supplements. Similarly, many conventional health care facilities offer *tai chi* or yoga classes through their existing exercise or fitness centers.

As with any organizational change movement, both attempted and successful integration efforts can instruct us and provide us with "lessons learned." Let us review a few such lessons below.

Typically, for these efforts to achieve even marginal success, it is necessary to have a "*physician champion*" for the cause of integration. As mentioned in the case description above, three oncologists were the driving force behind the integration of psycho-oncology services in the Hulston Cancer Center at Cox Health Systems. This is fairly typical of successful programs, in which a physician leader must bring together a "critical mass" of resources to meet the needs of a patient population facing chronic conditions. Indeed, it is often the awareness that patients are receiving these services elsewhere that provides an impetus for physicians and other decision makers to "pull them back in" to their care in an integrated setting. The physician champion must be a credible clinician with a good reputation and clinical skills, good communication skills, and the time and availability to conduct the project.

Advisory councils of key stakeholders, including physicians, health systems administrators, fitness center employees, nutritionists, psychologists, and various holistic practitioners, can help provide the direction and political muscle necessary for integrated efforts to succeed. The political and attitudinal barriers to integrating holistic care are high, and the boundaries often feel impenetrable. Appropriately constituted advisory councils can help to build consensus through continual data-based education.

When integration efforts involve *architectural design* and *construction* of offices or other facilities, it is crucial that the unique perspectives of holistic practitioners be considered. For example, the offices of psychologists, aromatherapists, massage therapists, acupuncturists, or chiropractors are likely to require very different atmospheres from those of family practice physicians. Such factors as color schemes, lighting, sound, and even smells should be thoroughly explored before expending too many resources on physical space integration.

Billing systems should be well conceived before attempting to "go live" with an integrated CAM effort. Such questions as whether to have combined or separate billing systems, and how to accept and process insurance claims for patients must be worked out. This is a particularly timely issue given that, at least in the USA, many insurance companies either offer or are planning to offer CAM benefits. For example, after extensive development of a network of accredited providers who are subject to quality assurance standards, Oxford Health Plan (U.S.) now offers a CAM program to members in several states. Mutual of Omaha has included Dr. Dean Ornish's heart disease reversal program in its coverage since 1993, and Blue Cross covers 50 percent of the cost of CAM therapies up to $500 per year in several states (cited in Kuhn, 1999). Why do such companies cover CAM benefits? The public demand for these services alone does not explain it. Insurance executive decision-makers are persuaded by the mounting scientific, clinical, and cost-effectiveness data supporting the inclusion of these holistically-oriented services.

The importance of the *selection* of the members of multi-disciplinary health care teams is another crucial lesson learned from integration attempts. Clearly, both providers of conventional and of more holistic treatments must be able to develop good working relationships with each other, for the benefit of their patients. Appropriate selection methods such as in-depth interviews, personality testing, and case reviews or analyses, pay dividends in fewer selection errors and better team facilitation. Interestingly, some CAM practitioners are reluctant to work with conventional physicians, rather than the reverse. Since CAM is a consumer driven movement, we should not underestimate conventional physicians' interests in working together in an integrated system of care. Clearly, practicing physicians feel more pressure to respond to CAM than do medical laboratory scientists.

Another too often ignored factor is precision in *defining the objectives* of the effort. It is crucial that both the medical system and the CAM practitioners be clear about the reasons motivating their integration, such as expanding the healing mission of the system, improving the reputation of the provider in the community, enhancing market share, and growing a new revenue stream. Only when objectives are understood can key indicators be developed and tracked to measure performance against these objectives. Conversely, when the focus and objectives of integration efforts are unclear, even minor operational difficulties can mushroom to derail an initiative in short order. Holistic initiatives are likely to fail if they are only reacting to a trend or because regional competitors are trying them. So it is all the more important that holistic approaches to health care are not "put in a box" at the periphery of the enterprise, but are incorporated into all of the acute and chronic treatment services delivered by the system.

Large-scale efforts at integration of CAM and conventional medicine are much more likely to fail or falter than are *smaller, incremental integration projects* that eventually achieve a "critical mass" within the system. As Thompson (2000) suggests, "The title of a 1973 book by economist Ernst Schumacher captures the essence of what's working today as hospitals and health systems try to bring alternative medicine into the fold of conventional healthcare: *Small is Beautiful: Economics as if People Mattered*. A modest scale also can aid the success of complementary medicine programs. And leadership from the people who matter—most notably conventional medical doctors—is proving to be pivotal in gaining support, trust and patient referrals."

Most health care systems have ongoing holistic services that are not part of some larger fabric of integration, and these same systems often have a tremendous unmet or unrecognized need for these holistic services. What is often needed is a mechanism or approach for bringing together the supply and demand for these services. At Cox Health Systems, one such effort, called the NOAH Project (which is an acronym for New Opportunities to Advance Health), is under way. A brief case description of this project may be illustrative of the problems and opportunities attendant to integration.

The NOAH Project maintains that: *it should be as easy for a doctor's office to schedule a patient for an educational opportunity, preventive services, or mind/body medical interventions, as it is to schedule a patient for an imaging procedure or lab work—particularly if similar offerings have been shown to reduce health care costs, enhance health outcomes, or dramatically improve patient satisfaction*. A system that achieves this goal can ameliorate the fragmentation, disruptions, and discontinuity of care often experienced by patients and providers in both managed care and more traditional health care arrangements. Such a system allows the original vision of integrated care—replete with prevention, health education, health-maintenance activities, and *strengthened partnerships between patients and providers*—to be more fully realized.

A *critical paradigm shift* is occurring—a shift into which health care systems can either lead or to which they will eventually be forced to adapt. Health care systems must increasingly embrace ways and means of maintaining health of those for whom they assume clinical responsibility. *The U.S. Preventive Services Task Force* (1996) *Guide to Clinical Preventive Services* noted the following points. (1) Conventional clinical activities (like diagnostic testing) may be of less value to patients than activities once considered outside the role of the hospital physician (like patient counseling and education). (2) One of the initial tasks of the physician practicing in this mode is shifting control to the patient. (3) Addressing the personal health practices of patients is among the most effective clinical interventions for reducing the incidence and severity of disease and disability. This report also emphasizes studies showing that clinicians often fail to provide recommended preventive services because of "inadequate reimbursement for preventive services, fragmentation of health care delivery, and insufficient time with patients to deliver the range of preventive services recommended." Mechanisms for correcting these problems, and for shifting more control to patients, represent opportunities for strengthening the patient-provider relationship.

Health maintenance organizations (HMOs), preferred provider organizations (PPOs), and other managed care organizations (MCOs) and the emergence of capitated systems of payment have brought dramatic changes for both providers and consumers of health care. While health care organizations once focused almost exclusively on helping people overcome illness or injury, on helping patients "get well," the focus is shifting to encompass both "get well" and "stay well" activities. Parallel to this shift in focus of providers has been a positive consumer interest in fitness, self-help, nutrition, health education, and alternative therapies. The stage has been set for a more dynamic partnership between health care providers and their patients.

Improvement in patient outcomes and cost-offset effects represent compelling reasons for the provision and coordination of a system-wide educational initiative for patients and families, including the outpatient population. Studies supporting this premise are voluminous, and cover nearly every major disease and disability known (e.g., asthma, arthritis, cancer, cardiac care, diabetes, etc.) In sum, the likely results of systematic, integrated provision of preventive, behavioral health, and health education services, coordinated through clinicians' offices are: *satisfied patients* with better health outcomes, more cost effective outcomes, and stronger affective attachments to providers and systems. In turn, enhanced provider satisfaction is yet another likely outcome.

While Cox Health Systems possessed a wide array of health education and preventive services, its physicians were not providing their patients with needed education and guidance regarding self-help, health maintenance, or complementary and alternative medical approaches. Although such services existed, physicians' offices neither advised patients of them nor scheduled patients for educational events. We simply lacked a systematic method for managing and coordinating the "supply" of education services with the "demand" or need on the part of physicians and patients.

In late 1998, the Burrell Foundation awarded Cox a grant to integrate its health education, preventive, and mind/body interventions with its other medical services. Principles and action plans are in place for the system-wide coordination of needs and resources through the NOAH Project. Working with an advisory committee of physicians, HMO case managers, psychologists, administrators, nurses, and information systems managers, the NOAH project coordinator coordinates supply and demand for alternative and complementary services. For example, physicians who have patients struggling with chronic diseases can now easily write a prescription for a variety of educational, preventive, and self-management services, including the very effective ongoing six-week Chronic Disease Self-Management Program (Lorig, et al., 1999), and the patient is quickly scheduled for this intervention. The initial outcomes from this wing of the NOAH Project are very encouraging; patients have shown significant increases in functional capacity on the SF-36 measure of health status.

The NOAH Project illustrates another important lesson from the struggle of integrating health care services. That is, many systems have "diamonds in their own backyards" that go unrecognized or undervalued until they are inventoried and placed in their proper contexts. Hence, it is often wise to begin integration efforts by focusing on what already exists within the system, rather than by looking elsewhere for needed skills and resources.

Conclusion

Having considered the driving and restraining forces surrounding integration of holism into conventional health care, we are left with many unanswered questions. Yet it is clear that health care in general and alternative medicine in particular face a series of critical decisions at this historical juncture. As Gruman (1997) put it: "Alternative medicine is at a fork in the road. [Holistic practitioners and scientists] should pursue scientific exploration of their services and should communicate their findings to fellow practitioners, but what they should do about becoming integrated within the mainstream health care delivery system remains an unanswered question. No matter where they practice, be it within conventional medicine, outside of it, or somewhere in the gray zone between the two, their work has the potential to contribute to the goals they share with the health community at large: the prevention of disease, the reduction of human suffering and improved health for all." Perhaps by focusing on these truly overarching goals, we can achieve a proper balance between the forces compelling and restraining the integration of holistic health care.

Acknowledgments

Preparation of this chapter was made possible by a research grant from the Burrell Foundation. Sincere thanks go to Dr. Todd Schaible, President and CEO of Burrell Behavioral Health, for his wise counsel and for reviewing early drafts of this chapter. Dr. Joe Hulgus also made helpful and insightful suggestions in the preparation of this chapter. Many thanks also go to Dr. C. Norman Shealy for his contagious commitment to truth and passion for wellness.

References

American Medical Association Council on Scientific Affairs. (1997). Report 12 of the Council on Scientific Affairs (A–97): *Alternative medicine*. Full text article available at www.ama-assn.org.

Astin, J. (1998). "Why patients use alternative medicine." *Journal of the American Medical Association*, 279, 1555–1561.

Barrett, S. (2000). "Be wary of 'alternative' health methods." Full text article available at www.quackwatch.com.

Chiles, J. A., Lambert, M.J., and Hatch, A.L. (1999). "The impact of psychological interventions on medical cost offset: A meta–analytic review." *Clinical Psychology: Science & Practice*, 6(2), 204–220.

Cohen, M. H. (1998). *Complementary and alternative medicine: Legal boundaries and regulatory perspectives*. Baltimore: Johns Hopkins University Press.

Dossey, L. (1998). "The Right Man syndrome: Skepticism and alternative medicine." *Alternative Therapies in Health and Medicine*, 4(3), 12–22.

Eddy, D. M. (1993). "From theory to practice: Three battles to watch in the 1990s." *Journal of the American Medical Association*, 270(4), 520–526.

Eisenberg, D., Davis, R., Ettner, S., et al. (1998). "Trends in alternative medicine use in the United States, 1990–1997." *Journal of the American Medical Association*, 279, 1569–1575.

Emerich, M. (1999). "Special report: New study defines $230 billion U.S. 'lifestyles of health and sustainability' industry." Article available at www.lohasjournal.com.

Fawzy, F. I., Fawzy, N. W., Arndt, L. A., and Pasnau, R.O. (1995). "Critical review of psychosocial interventions in cancer care." *Archives of General Psychiatry*, 52(2), 100–113.

Friedman, R., Sobel, D., Myers, P., Caudill, M., et al. (1995). "Behavioral medicine, clinical health psychology, and cost offset." *Health Psychology*, 14(6), 509–518.

Gruman, J. C. (1997). *Alternative medicine: Is it ready to join the mainstream?* Washington, DC: Center for the Advancement of Health.

Guide to Clinical Preventive Services: Report of the U.S. Preventive Services Task Force. (1996) 2nd edition, DHHS, Office of Disease Prevention and Health Promotion. New York: Williams & Wilkins.

Kuhn, M. A. (1999). *Complementary therapies for health care providers*. Philadelphia: Lippincott, Williams & Wilkins.

Landmark Healthcare. (1998). "The landmark report on public perceptions of alternative care." Summary available at www.landmarkhealthcare.com.

Lorig, K.R., Sobel, D. S., Stewart, A. L., Brown, Jr., B. W., Ritter, P. L., González, V.M., Laurent, D. D., and Holman, H.R. (1999). "Evidence suggesting that a chronic disease self-management program can improve health status while reducing utilization and costs: A randomized trial." *Medical Care*, 37(1), 5–14.

National Institutes of Health. (1994). *Alternative Medicine: Expanding Medical Horizons. A Report to the National Institutes of Health on Alternative Medical Systems and Practices in the United States*, (NIH pub. no. 94–066). Bethesda, MD: NIH.

Pert, C. B. (1997). *Molecules of emotion: Why you feel the way you feel*. New York: Scribner.

Shealy, C. N. (1980). "What is holistic medicine?" *Medical Tribune*, Jan. 23, 1–6.

Spiegel, D., Bloom, J. R., Kraemer, H. C., and Gottheil, E. (1989). "Effect of psychosocial treatment on survival of patients with metastatic breast cancer." *Lancet*, 2(8668), 888–891.

Thompson, E. (2000). "The alternative model." *Modern Healthcare*, 30 (20), 26–34.

Weil, A. (1995). *Spontaneous Healing*. New York: Fawcett Columbine.

Not Just Skin Deep

Treating Deeper Problems with Different Paradigms

4.
Acupuncture in the Modern World

Dan Kenner, L. Ac.

Introduction

Acupuncture is gradually gaining prominence as a health care modality in the modern world. The growth in popularity of such an ancient practice is a noteworthy phenomenon. The various health care practitioners who adopt the practice of acupuncture tend to have one of two basic orientations. "Classicists" view the traditions of acupuncture as sacrosanct and regard the classical literature of oriental medicine as holy scripture produced during a Golden Age of enlightenment. "Modernists" maintain that acupuncture derives from a paradigm whose principles provide a gateway to a future medicine more theoretically akin to modern physics than to biochemistry.

History and Background

It is well known that the use of acupuncture dates to antiquity. Acupuncture as a system first appeared in Chinese thought during the Han Dynasty (202 B.C.–220 A.D.), although there are references to the therapeutic use of needles in literature from earlier periods. As in many cultures, popular and folk medicine differed greatly from the elite medicine of literate doctors. Historically Chinese folk medicine centered around ancestral worship, propitiation of demonic forces, the use of amulets, talismans and herbal folk remedies. By contrast, a very small aristocratic minority practiced acupuncture. Because there is no written record except that of the literate class, we can only speculate about the role that needles played outside of this elite.

The Chinese medical classics, the *Huang Di Nei Jing* (second to first century B.C.) and the *Nan Jing* (first century A.D.) record the process of compiling conceptual features of Chinese medicine from earlier systems. These theories of evaluation and treatment developed as a quasi-system during the Han Dynasty. This is not to say that previous medical folk traditions died out at this time, but rather than medicine as a discipline began to separate itself from religion for the first time.

Acupuncture was represented in the *Nei Jing* as a medical modality resting on a theoretical foundation. The second volume of the *Nei Jing*, the *Ling Shu* is devoted almost entirely to acupuncture laws. By the time the *Nan Jing* was written, a more cohesive theoretical paradigm had emerged, including the diagnosis of pulse, a system of 14 main channels at the skin surface, and a method of regulating *qi* circulation in those channels based on traditional point classifications and established rules of treatment.

Acupuncture continued to develop during the next eras, the Three Kingdoms and the Six Dynasties. By the 6th century, during the latter Six Dynasties era, Chinese medicine theories and techniques had spread to Korea and Japan.[1] Vietnam has an even longer tradition of the use of acupuncture; the use of Chinese medicine in Vietnam may date back as far as the second century B.C.

The Sui Dynasty saw the reintroduction of religious ideas, this time particularly Buddhist and Taoist, to the practice of medicine. Although many psycho-spiritual elements remained even in the classical literature, "crossover" concepts such as the use of acupuncture to drive out demonic forces were introduced.[2] In the T'ang period, acupuncture theory did not develop significantly in China, but medical schools where acupuncture was taught were established.[3] Japan and Korea, however, witnessed wider growth and acceptance.

In the Sung Dynasty, neo-Confucian thought models established the *qi* energy paradigm as a scientific challenge to Buddhist metaphysics. This doctrine proposed *qi* as a type of universal vital force underlying all material manifestations and phenomena. Medical practice within this paradigm undertakes the regulation of the flow of *qi* as a primary objective. The scientism of the era attempted to create systematic methodologies for internal medicine based on Chinese phytotherapy and even Taoist and Buddhist exorcism. The primary developments in the Sung Dynasty were actually in the realm of phytotherapy rather than acupuncture.[4]

Although China came under Mongol rule in the Yuan Dynasty from 1264 to 1368, intellectual life was not suppressed, and traditional educational values persisted. Intellectual development of acupuncture also continued as new writings were joined by compilations of older classical materials. The *Nan Jing* not only survived as a classic of acupuncture for over a millennium but was even translated into Mongolian and Persian. Acupuncture was taught in medical schools along with moxibustion (heat treatment of acupuncture points by burning small cones of refined mugwort resin on them) and phytotherapy.[5]

During the Ming Dynasty, acupuncture reached its period of maximum diversity. Various schools of thought stratified physicians into different classes. Medical literature proliferated, including texts that were purely empirical such as the *Zhen Jiu Ju Ying* by Gao Wu. This was in some ways a golden age of Chinese medicine, but by the end of the era, the use of acupuncture had already begun its precipitous decline.[6]

The Qing Dynasty began with a period of peace and prosperity from the mid-seventeenth to the late eighteenth century, when the cultural flowering of the Ming Dynasty degenerated into a Babel of dissonance. Real masters of medicine became fewer and the *qi* paradigm lost dominance as a worldview.[7] The Qing period in China saw few influential medical texts written, but in 19th century Japan and Korea, there were numerous innovations in acupuncture and moxibustion. The Japanese acupuncturist Waichi Sugiyama introduced the use of the *shinkan*, or needle guide tube. The guide tube allowed the practitioner to easily use much thinner needles and freed one hand for point location and palpation.[8]

The influx of Western culture served to hasten the deterioration of the traditional Chinese philosophical underpinnings. Western concepts were adopted, but most of all the Western technologies played the dominant role in marginalizing East Asian cultural traditions. Western medicine had trickled into Japanese intellectual circles in the 18th century, and by the 19th century, dominated by anatomical studies and advancements in surgery and hygiene, Western medicine introduced a new materialism to the East. Japanese doctors studied the new sciences of nutrition and battlefield medicine in Bismarck's Germany, and on their return, they effectively banned traditional East Asian medicine. By the time of the First World War, acupuncture and Chinese traditional medicine faced cultural extinction throughout East Asia.

The Acupuncture Renaissance

Since its nadir at the turn of the 20th century, the practice of acupuncture barely maintained its existence until the end of World War II. During the years since then, its popularity and legitimacy have grown so phenomenally that acupuncture is now more widely practiced than at any time in its history. It is estimated that there are now between 1 and 1.5 million acupuncture practitioners in the world.[9]

In Meiji Era Japan, the practice of acupuncture was restricted to physicians trained in Western medicine. Acupuncture was seldom practiced openly. Among the few physicians using acupuncture, only acupuncture based on Western anatomy [the Dutch *Rampo* school of Gempaku Sugita] was tolerated as within the bounds of scientific theory. Traditional acupuncture, rooted in the *qi* paradigm, was eschewed. In the 1920s there was a backlash against the pure materialistic Westernization of traditional medicine by prominent figures like Sorei Yanagiya and Shinichiro Takeyama, who instigated a re-examination of the classical literature of oriental medicine. By 1930, empirical clinical evaluations of the classical literature had resulted in a call for a "return to the classics."[10]

By 1929, China had officially adopted Western medicine and prohibited traditional medicine. As a practical matter, China lacked both the financial and human resources to provide a Western-style medical system on anywhere near the scale required. In the 1920s, the *Zhong yi* (Chinese medicine) movement attempted to reformat and preserve traditional medicine in the hope of ensuring its survival. The *Zhong yi* movement's attempt to reconcile various schools and styles of traditional medicine later became the framework for the development of "Traditional Chinese Medicine" (TCM) in post-revolutionary communist China in the 1950s.[11]

The creation of TCM in post-World War II China was a way of providing adequate primary health care to a half-billion people of the world's most populous nation. Serving such a vast population with fewer than 40,000 Western physicians and over 500,000 diverse and disorganized traditional-style practitioners posed a colossal public health problem. Organizing and mobilizing an army of health care workers and developing a viable hospital and health care system was an achievement in social engineering of the first magnitude.[12] However, Communist China's materialistic bias toward Westernization became obvious. Less than one-third of Chinese medical schools have a traditional orientation. Western physicians now outnumber traditional practitioners two to one and make considerably higher salaries.[13]

The fact remains that traditional medicine, however altered, still plays a substantial role in Chinese health care today. By 1980, China had trained more than a million "barefoot doctors," the famous traditionally trained worker-practitioners. Today over 300,000 traditional-style practitioners have graduated from 5-year training programs in China's 24 medical schools.[14]

Acupuncture has grown into a recognized health care modality in the West as well. The number of treatments in the U.S. is estimated to exceed 12 million per year.[15] In the U.S. today, there are an estimated 11,000 licensed acupuncturists, of whom approximately 3000 are physicians. Over half of the states license acupuncturists, with varying requirements for licensure. In the U.K. there are no specific licensing requirements, but over 2000 practitioners according to one estimate.[16] There are physician and non-physician acupuncturists in the British Commonwealth countries of Canada, New Zealand, and Australia—over 4500 practitioners in Australia alone, an even higher concentration of practitioners than the U.S.[17] In France, acupuncture is considered to be a medical specialty. There are over 10,000 physicians trained in medical schools to practice acupuncture, although there are known to be a substantial number of non-physician practitioners.[18] Between 20,000 and 30,000 German physicians and 2000 *heilpraktikers* (natural medicine therapists) practice acupuncture.[19] In the Soviet bloc, acupuncture has been practiced in Russia and East European countries since the mid-1950s. Russian hospitals often practice acupuncture within "traditional medicine" departments.[20] Acupuncture is also practiced by thousands of physicians in Romania, Hungary, Czechoslovakia, Poland, and the former East Germany.[21]

The acceptance of acupuncture in the U.S. and the U.K. has resulted in insurance coverage for treatment even by non-physician acupuncturists in many cases. Insurance coverage in France and Germany for physicians practicing acupuncture has been available for several years. Insurance coverage in France, where acupuncture is a designated medical specialty, has resulted in an extraordinarily high rate of utilization, estimated at 20 percent of the French population.[22] As third party payment for acupuncture as a medical service increasingly becomes available, it is reasonable to expect that it will become more prominent as a mainstream medical modality.

Types of Acupuncture

The word "acupuncture" has become a generic term for a variety of practices that are used for diverse applications, and these applications are based on diverse theoretical paradigms. The following titles of research papers presented at a recent acupuncture symposium illustrate this diversity:[23]

"Does ß-endorphin modify the effects of acupuncture during anesthesia in dogs?"

"Can early detection of stomach carcinoma be achieved by *ryodoraku*?"

"'Wind' as a factor in pathogenesis"

"Acupuncture trigger point release for elbow tenosynovitis"

"Ultraweak photon emission from biological systems"

"Changes in the power spectrum of the EEG from moxibustion at sedation points"

"Influence of the 5 yin meridians on the dynamics of the peripheral circulation"

"Auricular ion pumping combination methodology"

"Low resistance acupuncture points in live and dead pigs"

There are four main types of acupuncture and numerous subtypes and schools of thought within these categories.[24]

The first type of acupuncture to have a large-scale impact in the West is *acupuncture anesthesia*. This technique was developed in the 1950s by the Chinese army for use in emergency surgery on the battlefield.[25] The widespread attention in the West to this type of acupuncture led to the idea that acupuncture is primarily effective for pain relief. It engendered the misconception that acupuncture gives instant pain relief, but is not therapeutic and only obscures the underlying problem. This argument was used to invalidate the use of acupuncture as a treatment for chronic pain when it was first becoming available in the U.S.

Conventional medical paradigms demand to know the biochemical mechanisms of new types of therapies before admitting them to the canon of legitimacy. Research at the University of Toronto elucidated that the body produces endogenous morphine-like substances, or "endorphins," that relieve pain and produce a sense of heightened well-being. The research showed that the pain-relieving effects of acupuncture could be attributed to the release of these endorphins resulting from needle stimulation.[26] This chemical "active principle" of acupuncture was the first step toward mainstream acknowledgment of acupuncture as a therapeutic modality.

Acupuncture anesthesia is not a true anesthesia, but analgesia, that can be combined with sedative and muscle-relaxing drugs. It offers tremendous benefits because of patients' rapid recovery times following surgery. There are also advantages in performing surgery on a conscious patient in some situations. The explanatory mechanisms include neurohumoral induction of a high level of endorphin release, combined with the effects of the strong needle stimulus creating a counter-irritation that interferes with other peripheral pain signals.[27]

The second type of acupuncture also uses fairly strong stimulation. *Acupuncture for physical therapy* relies on the use of motor points and trigger points that can motivate a neuromuscular interface, causing muscles to contract or relax. Trigger points can relieve tension in muscles and tendons that are hypertonic due to strain, injury or inflammation. The stimulation to the muscles or connective tissue can give a strong sensation and stimulate circulation, lymph drainage, and mobility of an affected area. Acupuncture performed for physical therapy relies on stimulating these points, but it would be premature to say that known physiological mechanisms are responsible for all such acupuncture effects.

A third type of acupuncture is known as *"meridian therapy."* Acupuncture meridians are the channels on which acupuncture points are located and through which the vital force known as "*qi*" is said to flow. The *qi* paradigm, as mentioned above, is the oldest explanatory model for the effects of acupuncture. The term *qi* is often translated as "energy." The idea of *qi* as energy is partly rooted in the post-Enlightenment concept of matter as something separate and divisible from energy. Evidence dictates that *qi* was considered to be a refined form of matter; "finest matter influences," as the German sinologist Paul Unschuld translated it. Its conceptual resemblance to the Vedic term *prana* and the Greek term *pneuma* is based on the connection between these terms and the idea of air as a vital source. In Chinese culture of the Han Dynasty, the concept of *qi* was a root concept with implications ranging far beyond its role in physiology and medicine. In the *qi* paradigm of acupuncture, *qi*, as a type of vital force, permeates the human body and flows along the acupuncture meridians and their internal pathways, which are said to connect to all of the internal organs and structures.[28]

The newer explanatory models show how China, Korea, and Japan came to value Western scientific concepts in the process of their modernization. From the mid-19th to early 20th centuries, many traditional values were discarded as part of an obsolete system of values and social organization, and even as superstition. The survival and modernization of acupuncture has resulted in new models that conform to Western paradigms of physiology and pathology.

The reductionistic approach to acupuncture has created a doctrine of "point specificity" in which single points are said to have specific attributes for treating specific diseases or symptoms. Likewise, clinical algorithms for specific diseases or symptoms have been developed as part of practitioner training curricula. This so-called "cookbook approach" to acupuncture is an East-West hybrid that purists claim bears no resemblance to the traditional methods that individualized treatment for each patient at each treatment session.[29] Curiously, this led to a "backlash"—a return to ancient concepts and methods not only in Western nations where acupuncture is a recent transplant, but also in Japan and Korea, where Western scientific values have been firmly entrenched for decades. The traditional frame of reference of acupuncture theory, including yin-yang and the five phases (often referred to as "the Five Elements": wood, fire, earth, metal and water), evoked a romantic attachment among acupuncture practitioners to its whole-system concepts opposing the reductionistic environment of conventional medicine.

The fourth type, *"homuncular" acupuncture,* conforms neither to classical notions nor to any modern scientific paradigm. A homunculus is a segment of the body that contains correspondences to every part of the whole; each subpart of the segment also has connections or reference to some analogous part of the whole. A common example used is a chart of the ear depicting therapeutic and even diagnostic points for the whole body. Points for treating problems of the hip, shoulder, and even internal organs such as the gall bladder or heart, are mapped onto the ear's topography.

Ear acupuncture, also called auricular medicine, was discovered and developed by Dr. Paul Nogier of Lyons, France in the 1950s.[30] In this conceptual framework, the ear is a fractal of the whole body in which, like a hologram, the whole is represented in the part. Dr. Nogier learned of a specific ear point that apparently relieved sciatic neuralgia. He speculated that the point had some type of correlation with the fifth lumbar segment of the spine, the origin of the sciatic nerve. Through a process of extrapolation, he derived points related to other spinal segments and by extension, other body regions. His clinical success using this model led to the development of auriculotherapy, the method of needling or cauterizing ear points for therapeutic effect. Auriculotherapy, also called ear acupuncture, has been developed further in China over the last 40 years.

Another example of homuncular acupuncture is hand acupuncture, developed in Korea by Dr. Tae Woo Yoo, in which points for treating the entire body are found on the hands. These new types of acupuncture have been the subject of very few research studies, and their underlying paradigmatic model is only hypothetical. The so-called "holographic" paradigm looks to nonlinear dynamics ("chaos" math) to explain distinct anatomical entities as "fractals" (units of self-similarity) of the larger organism.

What Is Acupuncture Used To Treat?

In the West, acupuncture earned its reputation for pain treatment because of the early interest in acupuncture analgesia in surgery. In East Asia, however, it has a much wider reputation for therapeutic value. The recorded history of acupuncture reveals treatments addressing a wide range of pathology, not just for pain relief or musculoskeletal disorders. Yet there are several problems inherent in evaluating this type of received knowledge. It is often difficult, for example, to ascertain precisely what was treated. Disease names are often translated from Chinese into Western languages as if a one-to-one correspondence existed between traditional and modern nosologies (categorization schemes), but this is hardly ever the case.

For example, Chinese medical dictionaries typically translate the term *dan du* (lit. "red lesions") as "erysipelas." In Chinese medicine, the term *dan du* can include numerous pathologies, including herpes zoster (shingles) that are not related to the life-threatening (Western) disease erysipelas, except that they also exhibit red skin lesions. The result of this type of inconsistency is to give the Chinese disease names and descriptions a false veneer of precision and translatability to the Western therapeutic context. This naive approach to translation also deprives Chinese medicine of its own voice with which to explicate its true complexity.[31]

Another problem in the body of historical literature on acupuncture lies in understanding how practitioners in earlier eras diagnosed patients. Evaluating a patient's condition was not based on the condition's alleged cause as much as by observable pathological phenomena: clinical signs. Using the erysipelas example, we can understand how red lesions on the skin were classified together as a group of clinical entities from which the subtype is selected by the diagnostician. In conventional medicine, red lesions would be a subset of a disease in which they occurred as a symptom.

In addition to its different methods of correlating symptoms and signs, conventional Western medicine is so heavily quantitative that non-quantifiable disease phenomena are considered psychological or even nonexistent. Traditional Eastern evaluation methods not only depend on sensitive observations by the practitioner, but value the patient's inputs and subjective experience in many diagnostic categories.[32]

Since Chinese medicine diagnoses patients into radically different categories than Western medicine does, it would be as ineffective as artificial to require the same acupuncture treatment for people with the "same" diseases in Western terms, without understanding the differences between their individual energy flows and needs. Typecasting patients into Western categories would completely ignore the advantages of acupuncture's tailoring of treatment to the individual's character and needs as diagnosed in the Chinese system.

So how can the clinical problems effectively treatable with acupuncture be determined? Standardized double-blind placebo-controlled clinical trials are not necessarily appropriate to this task. First, as we have just seen, Chinese diagnoses disagree with Western diagnoses about which groups of people have the "same" health problems, to the same degree, and for the same reasons. In administering treatment to the treated group, we should need to establish agreement on standardization of point locations and needling techniques. Is the best "controlled" acupuncture treatment one that uses mathematically identical locations, pressures, depths, and times for all patients, as Western "digital" medicine would suggest, or one that subtly adjusts locations, pressures, depths, and times according to the needs of the patient's bodily responses, as Eastern medicine would suggest? Finally, we would have to invent a "sham acupuncture" method in which needles were used in ways or places that were demonstrably ineffective or inappropriate, without other side-effects.

A better solution to obtaining more reliable information about the clinical efficacy of acupuncture is two-pronged. The first undertaking must be to use outcome research methods in clinical research. Outcome studies are clinical trials without placebo control. The effectiveness of a new treatment is compared to the effectiveness of other established treatments. Studies can even be performed in which acupuncture treatment is individualized for patients within certain guidelines, which would allow for a more "real life" approach to research.

The second undertaking must be to raise academic standards to train not only to read historical Chinese language medical texts, but with sufficient biomedical knowledge to understand Chinese medical terms both in their own contexts and in their relation to contemporary clinical approaches.

The difficulty of constructing medical research protocols does not invalidate the claims of practicing acupuncturists or the claims of the acupuncture tradition. The problem in medical research is to find a methodology that is appropriate for the modality in question. The answers to the question "what is acupuncture used to treat effectively?" are gradually beginning to appear. The U.S. National Institutes of Health (NIH) Consensus Development Conference panel on acupuncture agreed that there is substantial evidence that acupuncture is effective for pregnancy-associated nausea and vomiting, chemotherapy-associated nausea and vomiting, postoperative nausea and vomiting, and postoperative pain.

The NIH panel also called for further research on other conditions for which acupuncture is likely to be helpful, including headache, low back pain, fibromyalgia, myofascial pain, tennis elbow, osteoarthritis, carpal tunnel syndrome, addictions, stroke rehabilitation, menstrual cramps, and asthma.[33] Presentations to the U.S. Food and Drug Administration[34] and at acupuncture conferences in Germany[35] regard acupuncture treatment appropriate for chronic pain conditions such as neck pain, facial pain, knee pain, carpal tunnel syndrome, and reflex sympathetic dystrophy; and for acute pain conditions such as dental pain, postsurgical pain, and pain from invasive diagnostic procedures such as endoscopy and colonoscopy.

Acupuncture has also proven highly effective in treatment of substance abuse.[36] Originally acupuncture was found to be effective in relieving opiate addicts' symptoms. Later it was found that acupuncture could have a beneficial effect on other drug cravings. Recent studies have indicated efficacy for treatment of addictions and associated symptoms of alcoholism, cocaine dependence including crack cocaine, and heroin dependence. There is also evidence to support the use of acupuncture for depression.

Evidence also supports the use of acupuncture in cases of respiratory disease, breathlessness, asthma, and exercise-induced asthma-like symptoms. For neurological problems, acupuncture can be recommended for sequelae of stroke, paralysis, hand paresis, palsy, and Parkinson's disease. Among urological problems, kidney stone pain, bladder instability, and urgent, frequent urination are treatable. Gallstones and diarrhea are digestive complaints that are mentioned as indications. Obstetric and gynecological conditions for which acupuncture can be helpful include induction of labor, labor pain, breech presentation, and hormone imbalances including menopausal hormonal irregularity.[37]

Acupuncture does not have to be considered a primary treatment for these conditions; its role can be supportive. As a secondary treatment, the list could be even longer. For example, based on the endorphin hypothesis, acupuncture can readily improve optimism or a sense of well being in problems as diverse as traumatic injury and cancer. Acupuncture could conceivably be a useful secondary treatment for any kind of stress-related health problem.

How Does Acupuncture Work?

As suggested earlier, the mechanism of acupuncture depends on the type of acupuncture in question. It is likely that there are various mechanisms rather than just a single, chemical definition as the endorphin hypothesis proposes. The use of acupuncture as a trigger point therapy for muscle and joint problems is palpable and immediate. While the efficacy of following the meridian system, the *qi* paradigm, and homuncular acupuncture methods can be proven, this does not necessarily validate the entire paradigm that each system propounds.

Where there is a will to do so, modern technology provides new ways to investigate these Eastern paradigms. Devices like the superconducting quantum interference device (SQUID) could detect subtle changes in magnetic fields. Many researchers have found objective evidence of acupuncture meridians. Russian researchers have claimed to detect the meridians using electrical field interference. Researchers in France have visualized what they claim is a meridian using radioactive tracers. Chinese and Japanese experiments have measured energy outputs from the hands of masters of *qi gong*, a type of exercise used to strengthen *qi* in its practitioners.[38] Microphotoplethysmography research has enabled some interesting physiological studies on the effects of acupuncture treatment. Dr. Yoshio Manaka of Japan found that a minute needle stimulus in the lower leg of a rabbit consistently resulted in an increase in the amplitude of oscillation in the microcirculation observed with microphotoplethysmography.[39]

Experiments have shown that acupuncture can stimulate the discharge of gallstones. Acupuncture has been shown to successfully improve tonus of the urinary bladder to relieve incontinence. In recent research, single photon emission computed tomography (SPECT) was used to examine blood flow in the brain of human subjects prior to and following acupuncture. An increase in radiotracer uptake of nearly 20 percent was observed in the thalamus after acupuncture indicating enhanced blood flow to the midbrain.[40]

Studies using functional MRI imaging techniques have shown that parts of the cerebral cortex are activated by acupuncture stimulation of other points of the body. The specific areas of the brain cortex that are activated coincide with stimulation of relevant point locations based on traditional acupuncture literature. For example, the visual cortex of the brain was activated by stimulating a point on the lower leg traditionally associated with vision problems.[41]

Acupuncture has also been shown to have an anti-inflammatory effect. A study in which rats with inflammatory pain and edema were given acupuncture stimulation showed reduced inflammation and edema. Even reduction of swelling of an inflamed paw was observed in the acupuncture group. One mechanism of acupuncture that this study suggested was an inhibition of activity of neurons in the spine.[42]

In most cases it is not yet clear what is being measured, but there is sufficient evidence to overrule pure skepticism. Indeed, many vital processes still completely defy explanation, such as the upward movement of sap in trees with no heart to "pump" it, return of venous blood to the heart, and the complex development of embryos in utero, to name just three.

Outlook for the Future

The growth in popularity of acupuncture as a practice and as a profession in the U.S. has been astonishing, in view of the obstacles faced by other unorthodox health professions. The chiropractic and osteopathic professions were marginalized and reviled by conventional medicine for decades. Even today, the mainstream profession rarely acknowledges chiropractic, which is based on correcting structural problems in the body.

Osteopathy achieved acceptance through imitation. Today osteopaths in the U.S. have the status of physicians, perform surgery and administer prescription drugs, but those osteopaths who wish to specialize in the traditional osteopathic methods must seek special training.

The irony is that these methods emerged from the heartland

of the U.S. A corn farmer with an aching back would have preferred manual therapy for pain relief by a chiropractor or osteopath rather than be sedated with laudanum or some other pain killer prescribed by a "regular" physician. The hostile reception of such practical manual techniques can only be explained by examining the forces that control the medical marketplace, as Paul Thomlinson has done elsewhere in this volume.

By contrast, acupuncture—despite its *needles* (certainly the most anxiety-provoking aspect of day to day conventional medical practice), "inscrutable" oriental philosophy, and "mystical" forces (the qi paradigm)—was welcomed with relatively open arms. This can only be explained by a shift in the expectations and desires of health care consumers. In the 1980s, health care consumers in the U.S. began to embrace alternatives with great enthusiasm. A spirit of change began to affect the health care marketplace, which is still in the throes of radical reform if not revolution.

It is likely that the popularity of acupuncture will grow. In France, with third party payment coverage for acupuncture treatment, utilization is high, at 20 percent of the population compared with 1-6 percent elsewhere. Acupuncture will also become more visible in the U.S. as hospitals and HMOs (Health Maintenance Organizations, which combine an insurance plan with a medical facility where covered services are rendered) employ acupuncturists. Acupuncture as a profession is rapidly upgrading its standards, as the chiropractic and osteopathic professions were once forced to do for their survival.

Training of acupuncturists will probably also take place in more institutional settings, as is the case in China and in Japan, where acupuncturists often undergo internships on campus hospitals. This type of acupuncture training is available in medical institutions for physicians in Russia, France, and recently in Germany. American medical institutions will come to offer similar training as acupuncture becomes a more conspicuous feature of medical practice. Acupuncture will also become a prominent part of substance abuse programs in the U.S. and elsewhere.

Research in acupuncture is also gradually growing. In the U.S., NIH funding through the Office of Alternative Medicine gave acupuncture research an unprecedented legitimacy. Further efficacy trials will no doubt be carried out for a wide range of afflictions. It is also reasonable to expect that new research technologies such as MRI, SQUID, SPECT, and others mentioned above will foster research into new medical paradigms.

Just as Japanese doctors generated a backlash and a call for re-examination of the classical literature 50–60 years after their cultural moratorium on traditional ideas, the Chinese can reasonably be expected to do the same. Only look at the new recent Chinese research on *qi gong*. This type of research is also likely to interest new generations of doctors in the West, who are not so hypnotized by reductionistic materialistic paradigms. Research into subtle energies using devices like magnets and lasers on acupuncture points is easy to "blind" in controlled clinical trials. If the basic research can measure the physiological effects of such low-stimulus treatment methods, a new science of subtle energy medicine could develop in the 21st century. This type of research would go beyond uncovering how acupuncture works, to a new level of understanding the electrodynamic aspects of physiology.

Future research will graduate from efficacy research, asking "does it work?" and mechanism research, asking "how does it work?" to developmental research, asking how to use acupuncture to solve problems we can't currently solve. When acupuncture research reaches this level, it will approach real fruition as a medical modality and possibly as one part of a foundation for a new paradigm of biology and medicine.

Notes

1. Lu Gwei-Djen, Needham J., *Celestial Lancets: A History and Rationale of Acupuncture and Moxa*. Cambridge: Cambridge University Press, 1980, p. 263.

2. Unschuld, P. U., *Medicine in China: A History of Ideas*. Berkeley: University of California Press, 1985, p. 43.

3. Lu Gwei-Djen, Needham J., *Celestial Lancets*, p. 65.

4. Unschuld, P. U., *Medicine in China*, p. 165.

5. Lu Gwei-Djen, Needham J., *Celestial Lancets*, p.100.

6. Unschuld P. U., *Medicine in China*, p. 195.

7. Lu Gwei-Djen, Needham J., *Celestial Lancets*, p. 160.

8. Birch, S., Ida, J., *Japanese Acupuncture: A Clinical Guide*. Brookline, MA: Paradigm, 1998.

9. Ibid., p. 47.

10. Shudo, D., *Japanese Classical Acupuncture: Introduction to Meridian Therapy*. Seattle: Eastland Press, 1990.

11. Chace, C., Zhang T.L. (trans), *A Qin Bowei Anthology*. Brookline, MA: Paradigm, 1997.

12. Ibid., p. 66.

13. Rosenthal, M. M., *Health Care in the People's Republic of China: Moving Toward Modernization*. Boulder, CO: Westview, 1987, p. 172.

14. Evans, J. R., "Medical Education in China." In Bowers, J. Z., Hess, J. W., Sivin, N. (eds.), *Science and Medicine in Twentieth Century China: Research and Education*. Ann Arbor: Center for Chinese Studies, University of Michigan, 1988, p. 244.

15. Lytle C. D., "An overview of acupuncture." US Department of Health and Human Services, Public Health Service, Food and Drug Administration, Center for Devices and Radiological Health, 1993.

16. Thomas, K. J., Carr, J., Westlake, L., et al, "Use of nonorthodox and conventional health care in Great Britain." *British Medical Journal*, 1991 302: 207–210.

17. Bensoussan, A., Myers, S., T*owards a Safer Choice*. Macarthur: University of Western Sydney, 1997, p. 23.

18. Bossy J., (1993) "History and Present Status of Acupuncture in France." *Abstracts* of the Third World Conference on Acupuncture. World Federation of

Acupuncture and Moxibustion Societies, Kyoto, 1993.

19. Aldridge, D., (1990) "Pluralism of medical practice in West Germany." *Complementary Medicine Research*, 1990, 4(2): 14–15.

20. Rudenko, M., Kabaruchin, B., (1993) The System of Education in Traditional Chinese Medicine in Russia. *Abstracts* of the Third World Conference on Acupuncture. World Federation of Acupuncture and Moxibustion Societies, Kyoto, 1993.

21. Praznikov, V.P., "The Role of Acupuncture in Modern Medicine." *Abstracts* of the Third World Conference on Acupuncture. World Federation of Acupuncture and Moxibustion Societies, Kyoto, 1993.

22. Bouchayer, F., "Alternative medicines: A general approach to the French situation." *Complementary Medicine Research*, 1990, 4(2): 4–8.

23. *Abstracts* of the Third World Conference on Acupuncture. World Federation of Acupuncture and Moxibustion Societies, Kyoto, 1993.

24. Kenner, D., "A Taxonomy of Acupuncture." Proceedings of the First Symposium of the Society for Acupuncture Research. Society for Acupuncture Research, Bethesda, MD, 1994.

25. Chen, J. Y. P., "Acupuncture Anesthesia in the People's Republic of China." John E. Fogarty International Center for Advanced Study in the Health Sciences, U.S. Department of Health, Education and Welfare, National Institutes of Health, Washington, D.C., 1975.

26. Pomeranz, B., "Scientific research into acupuncture for the relief of pain." *Journal of Alternative and Complementary Medicine*, 1996, 2(1): 53–60.

27. Takeshige, C., "Mechanism of Acupuncture Analgesia Based on Animal Experiments." In: Pomeranz B., Stux G. (eds), *Scientific Bases of Acupuncture*. Berlin: Springer-Verlag, 1989, pp. 53–78.

28. Birch, S. J., Felt, R. L., *Understanding Acupuncture*, New York: Churchill-Livingstone, 1999, pp. 89–90.

29. O'Connor, J., Bensky, D., *Acupuncture: A Comprehensive Text*. Seattle: Eastland, 1981.

30. Nogier, P. F. M., *From Auriculotherapy to Auriculomedicine*. Saint-Ruffine: Maisonneuve, 1983.

31. Wiseman, N., *Glossary of Chinese Medical Terms and Acupuncture Points*. Brookline, MA: Paradigm, 1990, pp. xxvii–xxxi.

32. Birch, S. J., Felt, R. L., *Understanding Acupuncture*, New York: Churchill-Livingstone, 1999, pp. 189–193.

33. NIH, "Consensus development panel on acupuncture," *Journal of the American Medical Association*, 1998, 280(17): 1518–1524.

34. *Journal of Alternative and Complementary Medicine Special Supplement* 1996, 2(1).

35. Birch, S., Hammerschlag, R., *Acupuncture Efficacy*. New York: National Academy of Acupuncture and Oriental Medicine, 1996.

36. Califano, J. A., Kleber, H. D., *Center on Addiction and Substance Abuse Annual Report*. New York: Columbia University, 1992.

37. *Journal of Alternative and Complementary Medicine Special Supplement* 1996, 2(1).

38. Bi, A., Fang, J., Jiao, Q., Liu, X., "The effect of the outgoing qi on the expression of surface antigens on human peripheral lymphocytes," *2nd International Conference on Qi Gong*, Xian, 10–15 September 1989: 29.

39. Itaya, K., Manaka, Y., Ohkubo, C., Asano, M., "Effects of acupuncture needle application upon cutaneous microcirculation of rabbit ear lobe."*Acupuncture and Electro-therapeutics Research International Journal,* 1987, 12:45–51.

40. "Highlights of Research at the NIH Conference," *Newsletter of the California Society of Oriental Medicine*, 1998, 4(1), p. 5.

41. Cho, Z.H., et al, "New approach to the understanding of acupuncture using functional NM and possible explanation of the effects," *Clinical Acupuncture and Oriental Medicine.* 2000, 1 (2): 107.

42. Lao, L., Zhang, G., Wei, F., Berman, B., Ren, K., "Effect of electroacupuncture on hyperalgesia and fos protein expression in rats with persistent inflammation: A new animal model," *Clinical Acupuncture and Oriental Medicine*, 2000, 1 (2): 112–114.

5.

Successful Energetic Treatment of Chronic Depression

C. Norman Shealy, M.D., Ph.D. and
R. Paul Thomlinson, Ph.D.

Introduction

The use of electrical current in the treatment of illness and disease has been considered since antiquity (Jarzembski, 1985), and has appeared in the psychiatric literature since at least the early 1960s (Heath, 1963). However, it is only since the 1970s that appropriate devices for provision of stimulation currents have been available to clinical scientists for application and evaluation. Since that time, such devices have been used fairly extensively, with recent research demonstrating their safety and efficacy in improving attention and concentration (Southworth, 1999), short-term smoking cessation (Pickworth, Fant, Butschky, Goffman, et al., 1997), anxiety and other stress-related disorders (De Felice, 1997), headache, insomnia, and brain dysfunction (Klawansky, Yeung, Berkey, Shah, et al., 1995), and substance abuse (Jarzembski, 1985), among other clinical problems.

For 28 years, our work at the Shealy Wellness Center has focused primarily on individuals with chronic pain, virtually all of whom are also suffering from chronic depression. Over the last 11 years, we have evaluated more thoroughly the treatment of depression focusing upon that, rather than upon the pain itself. In 1975, we were introduced to a specific transcutaneous electrical nerve stimulator, at that time called the Pain Suppressor®. It later evolved into the Liss Cranial Stimulator, which can be seen in the photo below, named after its inventor, Dr. Saul Liss. In 1990, the Food and Drug Administration granted Dr. Liss authority to "market the device, subject to the general controls provisions of the Federal Food, Drug, and Cosmetic Act."

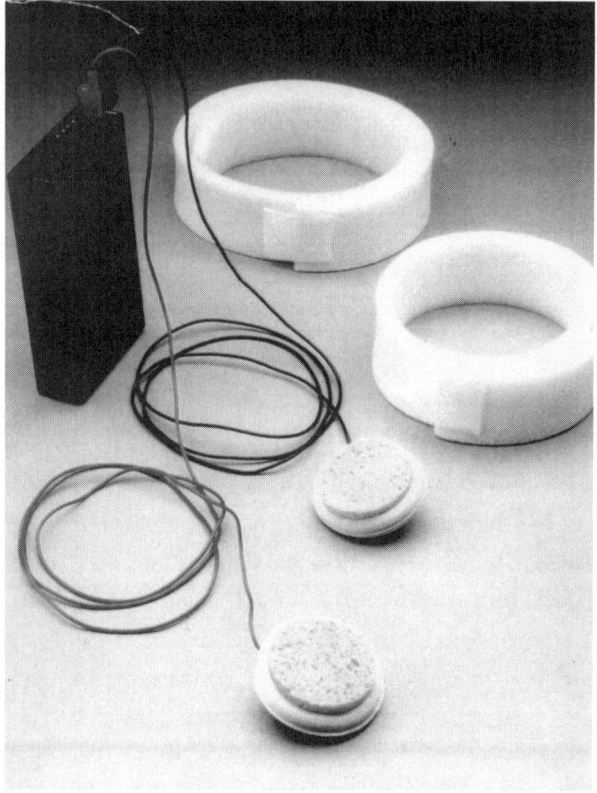

Liss Cranial Stimulator

Our earliest work with this device indicated that it had a striking ability to normalize total serotonin production (Shealy, Kwako, and Hughes, 1979). This finding has major implications for the application of cranial electrical stimulation (CES) to the treatment of a broad array of disorders, because "serotonin metabolism is disordered in a variety of clinical states, including both medical and mental disorders," and "potentially treatable low serotonin states are the final common pathway in many medical disorders" (Nash, 1996, p. 35). Indeed, it is not too strong to suggest that "an individual's genetically determined stable set point for serotonin may be disordered by environmentally induced events, leading to altered sleep, dysthymia, and depression. This imbalanced neurochemistry cascades into an autonomic nervous system hyperactivity causing symptoms" (*ibid*). Coupled with our own early work showing serotonin normalization from the CES, this "serotonin connection" inspired a long series of clinical studies, some of which will be reviewed in this chapter.

In the initial studies on this device, 40 percent of the patients were found to produce an excess of serotonin as measured by 24-hour output of 5-hydroxyindolacetic acid (5HIAA), and 40 percent had a deficiency in the production of serotonin (Shealy, Kwako, and Hughes, 1979). In both cases, application of the Liss stimulator transcranially normalized total serotonin production. Interestingly, those patients who had a normal 24-hour 5HIAA did not change their serotonin production and did not improve from any of the treatment modalities employed. In sum, it has been our experience for the last 24 years that the Liss stimulator applied transcranially is of particular value in normalizing serotonin production, and later studies have shown it to be effective when no other modality is used in at least 50 percent of people with chronic depression (e.g., Shealy, Cady, Wilkie, Cox, Liss, and Closson, 1989).

Its ideal use seems to be primarily to treat depression itself. The great advantage of this particular therapy is that with the exception of patients with cardiac pacemakers or implantable cardioverter defibrillators, there is no contraindication to its use, and indeed, these are purely theoretical contraindications. We have, on a number of occasions, checked patients with cardiac pacemakers while they were hooked up to their EKG and no adverse effects were found. Nevertheless, we do not recommend that one ordinarily use this type of stimulator in patients with pacemakers.

Research

Of considerable importance in looking at the broad field of chronic pain associated with depression, is the recent international study on the relation between somatic symptoms and depression (Simon, VonKorff, Piccinelli, Fullerton, and Ormel, 1999). It appears that in virtually all countries, depression is often either denied by the patient or masked when the patient seeks treatment of somatic symptoms rather than primarily of depression. Implications of this will be further explored later in this chapter.

According to Munoz, et al. (1994), "the majority of cases of clinical depression go unrecognized and untreated, despite the fact that depression is an eminently treatable disorder…" (p. 42). These authors go on to note that the recently published clinical practice guidelines from The Agency for Health Care Policy and Research (AHCPR), which focused on depression in primary care settings, "should enhance the detection of depression and the quality of psychotherapy for depression…however, the guidelines encourage primary care physicians to provide pharmacotherapy to their depressed patients as the first line of treatment" (p. 42). At the very least, as Munoz, et al. point out, "patients should be informed of the broad array of treatment options available and provided with a more balanced presentation of the potential benefits of psychotherapy for depression" (p. 42). Unfortunately, it appears that the AHCPR guidelines, data-based though they are, and their critics (e.g., Munoz, and others), well-intentioned though they are, both ignore a vast array of safe, efficacious alternative treatments that might loosely be grouped together as "holistic treatments for depression," including those described here. The remainder of this work will focus on CES as *one element of holistic treatment.*

Our clinical studies have involved some 15,000 patients with chronic pain and/or depression. It should be noted that all of the patients participating in the clinical research described here had been in depression for well over six months, all had failed one or more antidepressant drugs, and all refused or dropped out of psy-

Successful Energetic Treatment of Chronic Depression

chotherapy. Specific research studies purely on the neurochemistry and/or clinical effectiveness of the Liss stimulator applied transcranially have been done in over 1,000 patients. The next study done after that mentioned in the introduction (Shealy, Kwako, and Hughes, 1979) has not been previously reported. It was considered a pilot study at the time, and in 24 patients with chronic depression as measured by the Zung Depression Self-Rating Scale (Zung, 1965; Zung, 1973), patients were instructed in the use of the transcranial stimulator to use at home, with instructions to return two weeks later for a follow-up Zung Test and clinical evaluation. Twelve of these patients were out of depression with no treatment other than the Liss transcranial stimulator. When compared with the average antidepressant drug, this is a remarkably important observation; however, we have done considerable further testing.

One of our earliest neurochemical studies was on plasma catecholamines (Shealy, 1988a). 55 percent of 44 patients with chronic pain and depression had norepinephrine levels elevated above the upper limit of normal; one patient having some 500 percent of the upper limit of normal. Dopamine was elevated in only 12 percent of these patients, and standing norepinephrine levels were elevated above the upper limit of normal in 80 percent of these patients.

In another early neurochemical study (Shealy, 1988b), 42 of 80 patients had pre-treatment plasma beta-endorphin levels well below the lower limit of normal (2.2 picograms/ml). Normal levels for the standards are 4 to 10 picograms/ml. Nine control individuals without chronic pain and depression had normal plasma beta-endorphins. Six of the 80 patients had pre-treatment plasma beta-endorphin levels above the normal level, their average being 14.4 picograms/ml, and 30 more of the 80 patients had plasma beta-endorphin levels within the normal range. Following two weeks of intense therapy, the central component of which was the Liss cranial stimulator, the 6 patients with elevated plasma beta-endorphins remained elevated. All but one of those, however, with a low beta-endorphin level evidenced increased to normal levels.

Other studies have included measurements of plasma fasting levels of serotonin, beta-endorphin, norepinephrine, cholinesterase, as well as the ratios of norepinephrine to serotonin, norepinephrine to beta endorphin, norepinephrine to cholinesterase, serotonin to beta endorphin, and norepinephrine to the serotonin and beta endorphin ratio. Striking abnormalities were found in one or more of these tests in 92 percent of 14 chronically depressed patients who also had chronic pain (Shealy, Cady, Wilkie, Cox, Liss, and Clossen, 1989).

This research revealed that after two weeks of daily 20-minute applications of CES, 67 percent of the depressed patients showed improvements in their basic neurochemical profiles, and 60 percent had improved on the Zung Test by 9 points or more, with 50 percent of the depressed patients at that point having Zung Test scores below 50, indicating no depression. These findings are consistent with our previously noted research, which had shown a 50 percent improvement with cranial electrical stimulation.

Later research with 104 depressed patients indicated the same type of findings (Shealy, Cady, Veehoff, Houston, Burnetti, Cox, and Closson, 1992). Ninety-two percent of the depressed patients had one to seven neurochemical abnormalities such as those listed earlier. In addition, in another 200 patients with depression, 80 percent were found to be deficient in magnesium. All of 60 other depressed patients were found to be deficient in one or more essential amino acids, most commonly taurine. Another of our studies (Shealy, Cady, Cox, and Murrell, 1996) showed that, in 29 patients with chronic depression, 6 were clearly deficient (below the lab's range of "normal") and all of the others had DHEA levels below the average, except one patient with bipolar depression. Only two of these patients had levels of DHEA above the first quartile. Thus, 93 percent of these patients were in the lowest quartile of DHEA levels, or were clearly deficient.

In addition to these neurochemical studies, we have also looked at total symptomatology in relation to the Total Life Stress Score

(Shealy, 1984). The average patient we see has 49 chronic symptoms. Such elevated levels of emotional, chemical, and physical stress can be construed as either causes or consequences of significant dysfunction of the autonomic nervous system, and/or significant precursors of disease or illness. This symptomatic picture becomes extremely important in the assessment and treatment of depression, particularly in light of Simon, et al.'s (1999) international study of the relationship between somatic symptoms and depression. Particularly, depressed patients from a wide rangeof world cultures tend to report "somatic symptoms, such as headache, constipation, weakness, or back pain" (p. 1329), and varying degrees of somatization. Of particular interest to the present work is that many of these so-called somatization symptoms are well-suited for treatment with cranial electrical stimulation.

In our recent study of 351 patients with specific depression, 275 females and 76 males who had failed to respond to one or more antidepressant drugs were treated with a combination of 10 hours of educational lectures, daily CES with the Liss stimulator, vibratory music on the music bed with built-in speakers, and photostimulation at an average rate of 10 Hz (Shealy, Cady, and Cox, 1995). At the end of therapy over a two-week period with treatments only Monday through Friday, 85 percent of the patients were considerably less depressed, and three months later 70 percent remained improved without further intervention. Neurochemical abnormalities found in 90 percent of the patients pre-treatment were present in only 29 percent of those patients at three-month follow-up, and only 4 percent of the improved patients continued to have neurochemical abnormalities.

In a later study that has not yet been published, in 36 patients who were treated only with photostimulation, vibratory music, and an educational program, 58 percent improved on the Zung Test, falling to below clinical significance levels. This study highlights some of the other promising holistic modalities under investigation in our clinical research programs.

Thus, by way of summary of our clinical research findings, we can say that cranial electrical stimulation by itself appears to be effective in at least 50 percent of patients with chronic depression, both relieving their depression and markedly improving and normalizing their neurochemical profiles. If we use photostimulation, education and vibratory music for two weeks, we get 58 percent of patients out of their depression within two weeks. When we combine the photostimulation, education, and music with the Liss stimulator, 85 percent of the patients improve initially and 70 percent remain improved at three months without any further intervention. Obviously, much further and longer-term research needs to be done. However, it is our impression that the vast majority of our patients who have improved at three months remain improved up to two years later.

Clearly, though the focus of this paper is electrical stimulation, it is the integration of this modality with the other methods mentioned above, in addition to psychotherapy, nutritional therapy, exercise, and other therapies, that yields a truly holistic approach to the treatment of depression. More detail regarding the other energetic and holistic modalities used in this program is provided below.

Photostimulation

Photostimulation is done at a frequency of 1 to a maximum of 10 Hz with simultaneous lights into both eyes. Generally we have used a wide variety of photostimulators, but the most common one that we have used is the Shealy Relaxmate, which has been discussed in several publications (e.g., Cox, Shealy, Cady, & Liss, 1996; and Shealy, Cady, Veehoff, Burnetti-Atwell, Houston, & Cox, 1996). Patients are instructed to use this device for 15 minutes twice a day, and for one hour at bedtime.

The Vibratory Music Bed

The vibratory music bed contains speakers that allow patients to feel the music as well as to hear it. They are placed on these beds one hour per day during the two-week treatment program. The music we have chosen is either Beethoven's *6th Symphony*, Mozart's *Requiem*, Rachmaninoff's *Isle of the Dead*, Pachelbel's *Canon in D*, and/or Aeoliah's *Crystal Illumination*, the *Best of Kitaro*, Burns & Dexter's *Golden Voyage 4*, or Steven Halperin's *Spectrum Suite*. The patients are encouraged to continue listening to these when they go home.

Educational Lectures

Finally, patients have a total of 10 hours of lectures. The topics included are:

1. Health, Stress, and Psychoneuroimmunology
2. Physical Roots of Health
3. Nutritional Roots of Health
4. Attitudinal Health
5. Relaxation and Sensory Perception
6. Balancing Emotions
7. Sex and Sexuality
8. The Energetic Framework of Health
9. The Tribal Center
10. Sex, Power, and Money
11. Personal Power and Self Esteem
12. The Heart Center
13. Will and Power
14. The Mental Field
15. The Will Center
16. Spirituality Activating the Human Potential
17. The Transcendent Self

18. Healing
19. The Health-Wise Assurance Plan
20. Elegant Spirit

Interestingly, in one study we compared our videotaped lectures with live lectures. At a three-month follow-up, 68 percent of the patients who had the live lectures were still doing well compared with 80 percent of those who had the videotaped lectures. Furthermore, patients seem to remember more and ask more questions afterward when they had seen the videotaped lectures only once. So those patients did not have any more exposure to the lecture than the ones attending the live lectures. The live lectures always have a heavy emphasis on psychospiritual matters.

Standards

In our experience of using cranial electrical stimulation in well over 15,000 patients over the last 24 years, there have been no complications. An occasional patient has a very transient complaint of headache, dizziness or slight confusion. All of these cleared within an hour, and we are not aware of a single patient who has had any prolonged or serious complications or side effects of CES. In general, we use one to two milliamps of current, and the output of the Liss stimulator is 15,000 Hz modulated 15 times per second and 500 times per second. Although our work has been only bitemporal or nasion inion, there are many other transcranial possibilities that could be tried. Obviously, other frequencies might also be used, but we have no experience with those. The following table provides some of the technical specifications of the Liss device.

PARAMETER	NOMINAL VALUE +/- 10 %
Output amplitude into 1,000 ohms	*4 volts peak*
Rate	*15/500/15,000 hz*
Pulse Width	*33 microseconds*
Maximum Charge per Pulse	*13 microcoulombs*
On Time per Burst	*50 milliseconds*
Off Time per Burst	*16.7 milliseconds*
Power Source	*9 volt Alkaline Battery*
Contact Dimension	*Approx. 1.75 inch diameter*

Federal law in the United States requires that the Liss cranial electrical stimulator be used only by or on prescription from a physician. The specific federal labeling of the device is as follows: "Federal law [USA] restricts this device to sale by, or on the order of an M.D., D.O., or a D.C., licensed in the State in which he/she practices." Certainly as long as that requirement is in place, and considering not only our experience with 15,000 patients but many thousands by other practitioners, we know of no risk in the use of this modality. It is unfortunate that at the present time a psychologist or other health care practitioner cannot prescribe it.

The only two microcurrent stimulators available by prescription are the Liss stimulator and the Alpha Stim. We have no personal experience with the Alpha Stim in treating depression. However, we did try it in 10 patients in an attempt to raise DHEA by applying it to 12 specific acupuncture points and it failed to raise DHEA, whereas the Liss stimulator applied to these same acupuncture points significantly raised DHEA levels. Thus, we have preferred to work with the Liss stimulator.

It is important to emphasize that the Liss stimulator or the cranial electrical stimulator is very different from regular TENS devices used for treatment of pain. In general, TENS devices use a maximum output of 100 Hz and up to 60 to 80 milliamps of current, whereas the Liss stimulator uses a maximum of 4 milliamps (usually only one or two milliamps) at 15,000 Hz, as was mentioned above. Transcranially, we typically use a maximum of 2 milliamps. The pulses of 15,000 Hz are modulated by 15 Hz and 500 Hz, and it is apparently this very high frequency that allows the Liss current to be transmitted through bone.

Medical Education

Since psychologists and many other mental health practitioners are capable of working with patients with chronic depression, it certainly seems desirable that ways be found for them to use this most effective and simple therapeutic approach as part of their treatment repertoire. This is particularly true given the safety record of the devices in our and others' clinical research, and the two merely theoretical contraindications enumerated earlier (i.e., pacemakers and implantable defibrillators). Indeed it is our position that a one-day training session for any licensed mental health professional should be quite adequate for them to become proficient in the use of this particular modality.

Public Awareness

At the present time, cranial electrical stimulation is certainly underutilized in the entire field of mental health care, and most mental health professionals know only about the use of drugs or psychotherapy in the treatment of depression. It is critically important that patients and the public be made aware that cranial electrical stimulation is not in any way related to electroshock therapy or electroconvulsive therapy (ECT). Although some studies suggest that these much more drastic therapies may help 80 percent of severely impaired patients (Valente, 1991), the risk profile and potential adverse consequences of ECT put it in a completely different category of possible harmfulness than the cranial electrical stimulation advocated here. The stimulator is so safe that one can drive one's car while wearing it. Indeed, the first author has personally used it when traveling to and from Europe or the Orient, as its stabilizing effect upon serotonin is a tremendous adjunct in avoiding and minimizing jet lag. Additionally, it does not interfere during its application or immediately after with cognition or consciousness, nor does it require any monitoring during application. In our opinion, cranial electrical stimulation is emerging as the modality of choice for treatment of chronic depression, although when it is combined with photostimulation, education and vibratory music, it shows even more impressive outcomes.

Cost Effectiveness

The commercial retail cost of a cranial electrical stimulator is $980.00. We have stimulators that have been in use for over 15 years without any defect. In fact, the only major problem that we have seen is when one of the stimulators was inadvertently dropped into a tub of water. Then it had to be sent back to the factory.

Considering the fact that modern antidepressant drugs have a complication rate of 25 percent or greater and often cost $100 or more per month, the cost of the cranial electrical stimulator is clearly an advantage, because it is a once-in-a-lifetime purchase and can be used for many years, if necessary. Unfortunately, at the present time in the United States, third party carriers generally recognize this type of stimulation only for treatment of pain, and although it is approved for the treatment of anxiety and depression and insomnia, it is not generally covered by medical insurance. Nevertheless, its safety and efficacy make it a first choice in our treatment of depression.

Research Funding Issues

For the past 50 years, the vast majority of educational material which physicians receive post-residency is presented to them by pharmaceutical representatives. Similarly, most of the clinical research currently conducted in the U.S. is sponsored by the pharmaceutical industry. This industry spends $200 million or more in getting an individual drug to the marketplace, and a most noticeable trend is to directly advertise many of its prescription items to the public, often spending more on public advertisement than on physician advertisement. There is no competition from any non-pharmaceutical company. The pharmaceutical companies are clearly not interested in funding studies that compare non-pharmaceutical approaches to pharmaceutical approaches.

For many years, the standard antidepressant drug against which all others were compared has been amitriptyline. The average percentage of patients "recovered" after one week on amitryptiline has been around 40 percent. Some have argued that amitriptyline has a success rate of 80 percent in recovery from depression. However, that is 80 percent of those who completed the study. Twenty percent dropped out to start with. Thus, at best, 64 percent of those entering the program could be considered successful. Unfortunately, these studies often report even mild or minimal effects as "success." In addition, 78 percent had significant side effects of dry mouth, 75 percent drowsiness, 71 percent increased appetite, 65 percent dizziness, faintness or weakness, 62 percent craving for sweets, 59 percent constipation, 47 percent blurred vision, 44 percent tachycardia, 25 percent jitteriness, 31 percent nasal congestion, 31 percent nausea, 25 percent difficulty urinating, 25 percent excessive sweating, and 22 percent feelings of numbness or tingling. (Weissman, Lieb, Brusoff, & Bothwell, 1975). Contrast this with the remarkable absence of any such side effects with CES.

Modern antidepressant drugs, including Zoloft, Paxil, and Prozac, all are said to work by normalizing either the serotonin or adrenergic system. The complication rate with each of them is very similar to that with amitriptyline. According to *The Physician's Desk Reference* (1999), 41 percent of patients with Prozac had no change in their symptomatology and 23 percent were minimally improved. Thus, at best, only 36 percent were *much improved* or *very much improved*. Even at 60 mg. per day, a dose which is tolerated by very few patients and which increases complication rates significantly, Paxil led to only 44 percent of patients being *much improved* or *very much improved*.

The results with our combined therapy including cranial electrical stimulation, photostimulation, vibratory music and education yield results in patients who are *very much improved* or *much improved* at least twice as commonly as by either Paxil or Prozac. With all of the antidepressant drugs, 20 to 25 percent of patients had such severe "side effects" that they discontinued taking the drug. In addition to that, there is a huge percentage of other complications similar to those with Elavil or amitriptyline. Even using the Liss stimulator alone leads to very much improved and much improved patients in 50 percent of cases, and so is better than either Prozac or Paxil, with no significant side effects, complications, or high percentages of patients who drop out because of complications.

Availability

Further information about the Liss Cranial Stimulator is available through the Shealy Wellness Center at (417) 865-5940 (www.shealyhealthnet.com).

References

Cox, R.H., Shealy, C. N., Cady, R. K., and Liss, S. (1996). "Pain reduction and relaxation with brain wave synchronization (photostimulation)." *The Journal of Neurologic and Orthopaedic Medicine and Surgery*, 17(1), 32–34.

De Felice, E.A. (1997). "Cranial electrotherapy stimulation (CES) in the treatment of anxiety and other stress-related disorders: A review of controlled clinical trials." *Stress Medicine*, 13(1), 31–42.

Heath, R. G. (1963). "Electrical self-stimulation of the brain in man." *American Journal of Psychiatry*, 120(6), 571–577.

Jarzembski, W. B. (1985). "Electrical stimulation and substance abuse treatment." *Neurobehavioral Toxicology & Teratology*, 7(2), 119–123.

Klawansky, S., Yeung, A., Berkey, C., Shah, N., et al. (1995). "Meta-analysis of randomized controlled trials of cranial electrostimulation: Efficacy in treating selected psychological and physiological conditions." *Journal of Nervous & Mental Disease*, 183(7), 478–484.

Munoz, R. F., Hollon, S. D., McGrath, E., Rehm, L. P., et al. (1994). "On the AHCPR Depression in Primary Care guidelines: Further considerations for practitioners." *American Psychologist*, 49(1), 42–61.

Nash, R. A. (1996). "The serotonin connection." *The Journal of Orthomolecular Medicine*, 11(1), 35–44.

Pickworth, W. B., Fant, R. V., Butschky, M. F., Goffman, A. L., et al. (1997). "Evaluation of cranial electrostimulation therapy on short-term smoking cessation." *Biological Psychiatry*, 42(2), 116–121.

Shealy, C. N. (1984). "Total life stress and symptomatology." *Journal of Holistic Medicine*, 6(2), 112–129.

Shealy, C. N. (1988a). "Hyperadrenergia in chronic pain." *The Journal of Neurological & Orthopaedic Medicine & Surgery*, 9(2), 105–106.

Shealy, C. N. (1988b). "Plasma beta-endorphin levels in chronic pain patients at a comprehensive pain treatment center." *The Journal of Neurological & Orthopaedic Medicine & Surgery*, 9(3), 264–265.

Shealy, C. N., Cady, R. K., and Cox, R. H. (1995). "Pain, stress and depression: Psychoneurophysiology and therapy." *Stress Medicine*, 11, 75–77.

Shealy, C. N., Cady, R. K., Cox, R. H., and Murrell, M. (1996). "DHEA deficiency in patients with chronic pain and depression." *The Journal of Neurological & Orthopaedic Medicine & Surgery*, 17, 6.

Shealy, C. N., Cady, R. K., Veehoff, D., Burnetti, M., Houston, R., and Cox, R. H. (1996). "Effects of color photostimulation upon neurochemicals and neurohormones." *The Journal of Neurologic & Orthopaedic Medicine & Surgery*, 17(1), 95–96.

Shealy, C. N., Cady, R. K., Veehoff, D., Houston, R., Burnetti, M., Cox, R. H., and Closson, W. (1992). "The neurochemistry of depression." *American Journal of Pain Management*, 2(1), 13–16.

Shealy, C.N., Cady, R.K., Wilkie, R.G., Cox, R.H., Liss, S., and Closson, W.

(1989). "Depression: A diagnostic, neurochemical profile & therapy with cranial electrical stimulation (CES)." *The Journal of Neurological & Orthopaedic Medicine & Surgery*, 10(4), 319–321.

Shealy, C.N., Kwako, J.L., and Hughes, S. (1979). "Effects of transcranial neurostimulation upon mood and serotonin production: A preliminary report." *Il Dolore*, 1(1), 13–16.

Simon, G.E., VonKorff, M., Piccinelli, M., Fullerton, C., and Ormel, J. (1999). "An international study of the relation between somatic symptoms and depression." *The New England Journal of Medicine*, 341(18), 1329–1335.

Southworth, S. (1999). "A study of the effects of cranial electrical stimulation on attention and concentration." *Integrative Physiological & Behavioral Science*, 34(1), 43–53.

Valente, S.M. (1991). "Electroconvulsive Therapy." *Archives of Psychiatric Nursing*, 5(4), 223–228.

Weissman, M.M., Lieb, J., Brusoff, B., and Bothwell, S. (1975). "A double-blind trial of amaprotiline and amitriptyline in depressed out-patients." *Acta Psychiatrica Scandinavicum*, 52, 225–236.

Zung, W.W.K. (1965). "A self-rating depression scale." *Archives of General Psychiatry*, 12, 63–70.

Zung, W.W.K. (1973). "From art to science: The diagnosis and treatment of depression." *Archives of General Psychiatry*, 29, 328–337.

Not Just Smelling the Flowers

Acquiring Recognition for Aromatherapists

6.

Aromatherapy
Healing Aspects of Essential Oils

Gerry DePaula, M.D.

Introduction

What Is Aromatherapy?
Aromatherapy is the health-promoting use of essential oils (EOs) extracted from botanical sources. The extraction may be performed by steam or water distillation, cold-pressing (for citrus oils), or solvent extraction (primarily with carbon dioxide), the method appropriate to the plant material. Methods of administration include diffusion in air, direct inhalation, topical application, and ingestion. Health-promoting uses include all those beneficial to the physical body, mental and emotional states, and spiritual well-being, for indeed these cannot be separated from one another. However, this chapter here focuses primarily on physical health, as there is much less hard-core research available for the other aspects.

Some Preliminary Cautions

Essential oils are the most concentrated active botanical substrates that can be obtained from plants. Essential oils must be diluted in some fashion before they are used; even very small concentrations of essential oils can have significant effects, and more is rarely better.

Some people develop sensitivities or allergies to essential oils, in which case they should immediately cease and avoid using the EO to which they prove sensitive. This risk is heightened by the use of insufficiently diluted essential oils; cross-sensitivities may develop as many essential oils share similar constituents (Schaller, 1995). Some essential oils, particularly cold-pressed citrus oils, contain a constituent that changes with exposure to sunlight. This UV-modified constituent tends to produce sensitive reactions in users, so citrus oils must be used in low concentrations (usually less than 1 percent) to avoid sun sensitivity.

As essential oils are powerful botanical extracts, there is a risk of accidental poisoning if too much is ingested, applied topically, or inhaled. As with any other possibly toxic substance, essential oils need to be kept away from children. Although rarely fatal, accidental poisonings have occurred in children (Jacobs, 1994; Lee, 1997). When working with essential oils for extended periods, good ventilation is essential; this concerns not only manufacturers but also rebottlers and therapists, especially those using massage.

Another concern is the possible presence of pesticides concentrated in essential oils. There is an increasing interest in growing organic, pesticide-free plant material for essential oils, but this may not suffice to eliminate pesticide residues from essential oils grown on land that was heavily sprayed in earlier decades. Fractional distillation can remove pesticides, but this is not an option for small local growers and distillers, and it increases the cost of essential oils for everyone.

The last major concern is the adulteration of essential oils. Our growing scientific understanding of the chemistry of these oils increases the opportunities to adulterate essential oils in ways that can be hard to detect. Sometimes a particular substance, e.g. linalool, may be added to an EO such as lavender to "standardize" it, i.e. to diminish variations from year to year or crop to crop. If sprayed on the plant material before distillation, it can be said that nothing were added to the EO from the time it came from the still. Sometimes adulteration can be detected because some plants make particular unequal ratios of chiral molecules, mirror images of each other. Adulterants fabricated in the laboratory usually display even mixtures of (+) and (-) molecules, that alter the expected ratio of these chiral components in the EO. Of course modern laboratory techniques can separate these chiral variations, but except for the most expensive essential oils, this is rarely economically feasible.

Other more obvious adulterations have gone on for decades. Some manufacturers allow their absolutes to contain unacceptably high levels of hexane solvents. Others dilute the pure EO with natural carriers like jojoba, almond, or even coconut oil, or with synthetic carriers like isopropyl myristate, yet sell their diluted products as "pure" essential oils. Experts can detect these adulterations by smell or by observing carrier residues. Even beginners can discover many carrier-oil adulterations by testing a tiny sample of the oil on a fabric such as silk and washing the sample; essential oils will wash out cleanly, but most carrier oils will not.

The Benefits of Essential Oils

There are many reasons for essential oils' age-old popularity in pharmacopeia. Essential oils are extracted from their botanical sources at their peak. The ratio of EO to plant material is small, so essential oils efficiently condense the biologically active components of plants for transport and storage. In their concentrated state, essential oils do not tolerate bacterial, viral or fungal growth (Maudsley, 1999), so they are not prone to spoilage. Kept in glass bottles, they are not exposed to vermin infestation like their fresh or dried plant source materials (Brandao, 1998). Glass bottles also minimize oxidation, particularly if dark colored or stored away from light.

Since essential oils are normally distilled in the geographical area where the plants grow, this usually keeps the costs very modest for local use. International transportation and national import duties raise their costs somewhat, yet the cost of many essential oils is still quite modest compared to other pharmaceuticals.

Holistic healing recognizes that the body possesses many methods and mechanisms for healing. When a natural form of healing is working well, intervention is minimal, just enough to stimulate the body's own healing mechanisms. When more than that is done, the intervention risks throwing the body out of balance, perhaps worse than the illness or malady needing care in the first place. One example of this is clearly illustrated by an elderly patient of mine who had osteoarthritis, especially in her knees. Her doctor placed her on a non-steroidal anti-inflammatory drug (NSAID) to help with her pain and inflammation, but that created a stomach upset. Then he prescribed a histamine blocking, anti-ulcer drug to overcome her stomach upset. This drug made her so light-headed and dizzy that she became fearful of falling and breaking a hip.

After consultation about aromatherapy, we agreed to use a blend of anti-inflammatory essential oils in a cream base applied topically to her knees two or three times a day. This afforded enough pain relief that she could decrease her NSAIDs by more than half. This allowed her to stop the anti-ulcer drug, and her lightheadedness disappeared. With continued use of the cream, she was able to maintain low pain levels, enjoy increased activity, mobility, and sense of well-being while using a minimum of NSAIDs. The essential oils selected for her had not only anti-inflammatory action, but they were mentally stimulating and pleasantly scented. She enjoyed these added side benefits, particularly compared to the adverse side effects she had just endured. This now happier patient was not only saving money on her medical treatment, but felt more involved in her own care, further contributing to her sense of well-being.

Research

Based on the above definition, aromatherapy is suited for healing people of all ages, races, and cultures. It can be used to treat a wide range of symptoms and conditions. As this chapter cannot include every use of every essential oil, we shall highlight research on three areas of essential oil (EO) use: (1) antimicrobial effects; (2) anti-inflammatory/analgesic effects; (3) metabolic effects of essential oils.

(1) Antimicrobial Action of Essential Oils

Recent laboratory evidence of the anti-bacterial properties of essential oils substantiates folk knowledge about plant oils used around the world for hundreds of years. Ross (1980) and many followers have conducted laboratory studies on the efficacy of essential oils and their constituents inhibiting the growth of bacteria. Currently, laboratory studies from Australia, Brazil, Canada, China, England, France, Greece, India, Italy, Japan, Kenya, Korea, Scotland, South Africa, Spain, Turkey, the USA, Zaire, and more confirm such folk knowledge.

Several aspects of essential oils complicate these studies. First, the ratios and concentrations of EO constituents vary not only from year to year, but also with place of origin and exact method of distillation. Second, while essential oils are volatile at room temperature, they are insoluble in water. This makes them more difficult to test in the laboratory, yet contributes to their mode of action, particularly on lipophilic cell membranes, as we will see in a moment.

Studies have been done with a wide range of essential oils on a wide range of both Gram positive and Gram negative bacteria. [Bacteria stained by the Gram method either pick up the stain (+) or they do not (-); this is a common method used in bacterial identification.] In general, bacteria are selected for study because they lead to food spoilage or poisoning, are common human or plant pathogens, or have developed antibiotic resistance. In general, essential oils are more effective in inhibiting growth of Gram positive bacteria than Gram negative bacteria.

Most research employs one of two laboratory methods to measure the efficacy of essential oils against bacteria. The first method uses agar dishes plated with known bacteria as its medium. The EO is placed on 5–7 mm. round discs, and the zone of inhibited growth around the impregnated discs (varying with the EO and concentration) shows the effectiveness of the EO. The second uses a broth as the culture medium. A known bacterium and a known EO at a specific concentration are added. Turbidity is measured after a specific amount of time and compared to controls; the more turbid the broth, the higher the concentration of bacteria.

Some of the many essential oils that have proven successful in such experiments inhibiting bacterial growth include: *Cistus creticus, Cymbopogon densiflorus,* other *Cymbopogon* varieties, *Helichrysum amorginum, Helichrysum italicum, Lavendula officinalis, Melaleuca alternifolia, Melissa officinalis, Ocimum basilicum linalool, Ocimum basilicum methyl chavicol, Rosemarinus officinalis, Thymus capitus* and *Thymus vulgaris.* Other studies identify the essential oils used by their common names: citronella, eucalyptus, geranium, orange, palmarosa, patchouli, peppermint and so on. (This difference in styles of reporting botanical names vs. common names makes it more difficult to compare studies and to compile good review data. The botanical name is more precise; a common name may refer to more than one plant; they are not always equivalent. The studies most useful for comparisons use both names; hopefully, this will become the standard for future studies.)

Not all the studies use the same bacteria, but certain trends emerge. Mangena (1999) found his South African Rosemary effective against salmonella, shigella, and staphylococci, among others. Pattniak (1996) found his Indian eucalyptus, lemongrass, orange, and peppermint effective against 22 of 22 different bacteria, aegle and palmarosa effective against 21 of 22, and ageratum and patchouli effective against 20 of 22. Wan (1998) worked with two varieties of *Basil-linalool* (BL) and *-methyl chavicol* (BMC). He found them effective against numerous bacteria except for *Clostridium sporogenes, Flavimonas oryzihabitans* and three species of *Pseudomonas.* (*Pseudomonas* prove even more resistant to essential oils than antibiotic-resistant *Staphylococcus aureus* in the concentrations that inhibited most other tested bacteria. Pattniak (1995) found *Pseudomonas aeruginosa* VR-6 resistant to all his tested essential oils at 20 microliters/ml. concentration.)

Impressed by the effectiveness of essential oils in inhibiting bacterial growth, many researchers have sought to find the active constituents of essential oils. Pattniak (1997) found cineol inhibited 16 of 18 bacteria; citral, 14 of 18; geranial, 16 of 18; linalool, 17 of 18; and menthol, 15 of 18. Chinou (1996) reported his *Helichrysums* were composed mainly of geraniol, geranyl acetate, neryl acetate, and nerolidol, but did not test these constituents individually. Mangena (1999) suggested camphene and alpha-pinene were particularly effective. Tirillini (1996), in his study of *Piper augustifolium*, suggested that camphor and camphene were the active constituents. Working with *Cistus creticus subsp. creticus* against *Staphylococcus aureus, S. epidermidis* and *S. hominis*, Demetzos (1999) found diterpene sclareol was the effective component.

In our modern world of high antibiotic use, we are interested in antibiotic resistant *Staphylococcus aureus*. Carson, Cookson, et al (1995) studied 66 isolates of *S. aureus* with *Melaleuca alternifolia*, also known as Tea Tree Oil (TTO). They found 64 of 66 isolates of S. aureus were methicillin resistant and 33/66 were mupirocin resistant, yet 66/66 were susceptible to TTO. Here the mean inhibitory concentration (MIC) was 0.25 percent and the mean bactericidal concentration (MBC) was 0.5 percent. Their British collaborators found comparable results in their *S. aureus* strains. In studying the major components of Tea Tree Oil, Carson and Riley (1995) found 1-terpinene-4-ol most effective, with linalool and alpha-terpineol very close seconds. (Again, the resisters were *Pseudomonas*.)

The Mechanisms of Antimicrobial Essential Oils

Takaisu-Kikuni (1996), studying the effects of *Cymbopogon densiflorus* on *Staphylococcus aureus*, found that high doses impaired growth in a bacteriostatic manner (like chloramphenicol), while low doses caused an energy/heat loss that caused the bacterial cell metabolism to become ineffective. Ultrastructure studies showed cell morphology changes characteristic of bactericidal antibiotics (like penicillin), causing bacteriolysis, or rupture of the bacterial cell membrane that kills the bacteria. This showed that essential oils can have both bacteriostatic and bactericidal action. This study also suggested that essential oils may have anti-bacterial activity specifically on cytoplasmic and cell wall metabolism.

Cox (1998) studied some of the active constituents of *Melaleuca alternifolia* (TTO) against *Escheria coli*. He studied 1-terpinene-4-ol, alpha-pinene, linalool, and alpha-terpineol. He found that terpenes accumulate in lysosome membranes, causing loss of membrane integrity and dissipation of the proton motive force. He found that at 0.5 percent TTO respiration in the exponential (multiplication) phase cell suspensions was completely inhibited, and that in the stationary (resting) phase cell suspensions it was partially inhibited. Naturally, the death rate of cells was higher in the exponential phase cells. Cox (1998) also studied whole TTO, to further investigate its action on membrane functions and cell respiration of *E. coli*. He measured oxygen consumption as a reflection of glucose-dependent respiration and K+ ion concentration as a measure of K+ leakage from cells in both exponential and stationary phases. (Healthy cell membranes maintain a high K+ concentration inside the cells; leakage indicates failing membrane function.) He found that 0.5 percent TTO (2xMBC) completely inhibited respiration in the exponential phase and decreased it to 43 percent of control in the stationary phase. When 0.25 percent and 0.5 percent TTO were added to exponential and stationary phase cells, K+ leakage began within one minute, but was slower in stationary phase cells. He concluded that TTO kills bacteria in a manner similar to membrane-active disinfectants.

Gustafson (1998) also studied TTO (whole oil) with *E. coli*. He found that TTO stimulates autolysis in exponential and stationary phase cells. Electron micrographs of cells grown in the presence of TTO showed loss of electron dense material, coagulation of cell cytoplasm, and formation of extra-cellular blebs. This was more pronounced in the exponential phase cells. In the stationary phase cells, Gustafson found less autolysis, but a sub-population of stationary phase cells demonstrated increased tolerance to TTO's bactericidal effects. This is an important finding as it raises the question of whether bacteria can possibly develop resistance to essential oils as they do to antibiotics.

Hamner (1999) did a study of TTO inhibiting growth of various organisms under conditions that might be encountered outside the laboratory. He found that 1 percent TTO and organic matter compromised the concentration of TTO it took to inhibit growth of *S. aureus* and *Candida albicans*. 10 percent TTO plus organic matter compromised activity against *Pseudomonas aeruginosa*. Organic matter affected 1 percent and 2 percent TTO, but not 4 percent and 8 percent, against *E. coli*. Hamner also measured surfactants and found that they too disrupt the anti-microbial activity of TTO, although the degree of disruption varies with organisms.

Soderberg (1996) alarmed aromatherapists when he reported on the toxicity of conifer resin acids (known cytotoxins), a tapped resin from *Pinus merkusii*, and TTO on epithelial cells and fibroblasts. (Epithelial cells are skin cells, and fibroblasts are present in and necessary for all wound healing.) A careful reading of his paper reaffirms the toxicity of the conifer resin acids, and the pine resin, but TTO only in concentrations above 30 percent. We should remember the toxicity of TTO in concentrations above 30 percent on epithelial cells and fibroblasts before we use TTO undiluted on the skin or wounds. As noted earlier, 0.25 percent to 0.5 percent proved bacteriocidal, depending upon researcher and laboratory.

Whole conifer resins are little used in aromatherapy because they are known sensitizers. In aromatherapy, conifer essential oils are generally distilled from the needles or sometimes distilled from the resin. This practice eliminates most of the risks of sensitization in using conifer essential oils. Soderberg (1996) mentions one significant risk that "...abietic acid, one of the main components from conifer oleoresin, has been shown to cause lysis of alveolar epithelial cells and is suggested responsible for the asthmatic reactions occurring in some wood workers."

Antimicrobial Action of Essential Oils: Anti-Fungal Section

Given the the time-honored use of culinary herbs and spices, along with recent laboratory demonstration of the anti-bacterial action of essential oils, it should be no surprise that research shows essential oils prevent food spoilage. Outtara (1997), Lachowicz (1998), Smith-Palmer (1998) and many others present convincing evidence that essential oils will likely have an increasing role as food preservatives. In addition to those studies, some have focused upon specific fungi. Caccioni (1998) studied citrus fruit essential oils and constituents on the growth of *Penicillum digitatum* and *P. italicum*. He found that the monoterpenes, except for limonene, and the susquiterpene constituents correlated positively with inhibiting pathogenic fungi growth. Of his group, citron and lemon essential oils performed the best. Pattniak (1996) used the same essential oils that he had tested against bacteria against 12 fungi: 3 yeast-like and 9 filamentous. He found aegle, citronella, geranium, lemongrass, orange, palmarosa and patchouli effective in inhibiting growth of 12 of 12 fungi; peppermint and eucalyptus worked with 11 of 12, but ageratum inhibited only 4 of 12. He then studied the constituents of these essential oils against the 12 fungi (1997). He found citral and geraniol best (12/12), linalool next (11/12) and cineol and menthol following (7/12). While some essential oils are both bactericidal and fungicidal, it is not necessarily the same constituents working in both instances.

So preserving the safety of edible food stores is one valuable use of essential oils. Further evidence suggests that essential oils are not only useful to prevent spoilage, but have fewer side-effects and potentially greater cost-benefit than traditional post-harvest fungicides. Mishra (1994) screened *Cymbopogon citratus* for antifungal activity against *Aspergillus flavus* in stored feed, discovering a wide fungitoxic spectrum, non-phytotoxic nature and superiority over synthetic fungicides. Mishra concluded that its fungitoxic potency remained unaltered over 7 months, even upon introduction of high doses of inoculum of test fungi, and remained thermostable from 5 to 100°C. Also working with *A. flavus*, Mahmoud (1994) measured the production of aflatoxin, the deadly and highly carcinogenic toxin produced by this fungus. Using aerosol essential oils, Mahmoud found that thymol (200 ppm), cinnamaldehyde (250 ppm), geraniol, nerol, and citronellol (500 ppm) all suppressed aflatoxin production as well as *A. flavus* growth. He found that citral, citronellol and eugenol prevented fungal growth and toxin formation for up to 8 days, although after 15 days the toxin production exceeded controls. Such studies indicate that further research is desirable to confirm the best methods of EO application and duration of anti-fungal activity, but they suggest safe and inexpensive ways to protect stores of peanuts, wheat, rice corn and other grains from attack by *A. flavus* and contamination by aflatoxin.

In addition to protecting food from fungal contamination, essential oils can effectively treat human fungal infections as well. For example, AIDS patients are often threatened by gastro-intestinal fungal infections of *Cryptococcus neoformans*, but evidence suggests that essential oils may effectively control such infections. Viollon (1994) studied the activities of essential oils and their constituents against the fungus *Cryptococcus neoformans*, originally obtained from an HIV patient. She found essential oils of palmarosa, clove, origanum, savory, tea tree, thyme, geranium and cinnamon had the lowest minimum fungicidal concentrations (MFC), all 400 microliters per liter or less. Of the constituents she tested, thymol (MFC = 50 microliters per liter), carvacrol (100), citral, citronellol (150), geraniol, beta-ionone (200), carvone, eugenol, farnesol, cis-jasmone and nerol (400) were the most effective against this fungus. This is helpful information to guide us in treating immune-compromised patients who can die from this gastro-intestinal fungal infection.

Vaginal herpes and related skin problems can also be ameliorated using essential oils. Suresh (1997) studied the essential oil of *Santolina chamaecyparissus* (MIC = 62.5–125 micrograms/ml) against *Candida albicans*. After he found it effective to inhibit growth of the fungus, he tested it *in vivo* in mice and guinea pigs against a standard drug treatment. He tested a 4 percent EO compared to 2 percent clotrimazole p.v., treating induced *Candida* vaginal infection. Although the EO took a little longer to work, the two treatments proved equally effective. He also compared EO with ketoconazole, both 60 mg/kg, p.o., against induced systemic candidosis. The survival rate was better for the ketoconazole (both were much better than controls), but the growth of fungi from harvested organs showed better results for the EO treatment. When he inoculated guinea pigs dermally to infect their hair roots, and treated them with 4 percent EO or 2 percent clotrimazole, clinically they showed the same improvement. Suresh's studies show that essential oils can be as effective as standard clinical prescriptions, with less toxicity and fewer side effects than the standard!

Tea tree oil has proven effective against sub-cuticle and nail bed fungal infections. Buck (1994) treated 117 patients with onychomycosis (under-nail, nail bed fungal infection) confirmed by culture, with either TTO (100 percent concentration) or clotrimazole (1 percent solution). At the end of six months, after twice daily treatment and debridement at 0, 1, 3, and 6 months, clinical assessment showed essentially the same rate of cure (60-61 percent) for tea tree oil as for 1 percent clotrimazole, while TTO had a greater rate of extinguishing the fungus completely (18 percent) than did clotrimazole (11 percent). Three months later, those showing continued improvement or resolution was 55 percent for those using clotrimazole and 56 percent using TTO. Against the same infection, Syed (1999) tested a cream combining 2 percent butenafine HCl and 5 percent TTO (vs. placebo) in 60 patients. He found an 80 percent cure rate in his treatment group after 16 weeks. At follow up, there was no relapse in the cured group and no improvement in the treatment resistant or placebo groups. This suggests that if a treatment has not worked over four months, another compound should be tried.

A wide variety of fungal infections of mucous membranes and the skin, including chronic dandruff, can also be controlled using essential oils. Lima (1993) tested 13 essential oils against dermatophytes isolated from symptomatic patients. Of his Brazilian essential oils tested, *Cinnamomum zeylanicum, Ocimum gratissimum, Eugenia uniflora, Alpinia speciosa, Cymbopogon citratus, Acanthospermum hispidum* and *Pneumus boldus* inhibited a great majority of test organisms. Nenoff (1996) tested for MIC for 26 strains of dermatophyte species, 54 yeasts (including 32 strains of *C. albicans*) and 22 *Malassezia furfur* strains. After determining the geometric mean MIC for these 3 groups, he concluded that TTO ointment should be used *in vivo* against fungal infections of the skin and mucous membranes and against chronic or fungal dandruff.

(2) Anti-inflammatory Action of Essential Oils

In order to understand the anti-inflammatory and analgesic actions of essential oils, it is helpful to understand some of the body's inflammatory responses. One immediate inflammatory reaction is mediated by histamine release, primarily from mast cells. This often instigates the formation of prostaglandins (PG) and leukotrienes (LT). Prostaglandins (PGs) have many functions in the body, with the number and position of double bonds and hydroxyl groups determining the physiologic properties of the various PGs. Even in very low concentrations, "inflammatory" PGs cause increased permeability of capillaries, loss of plasma proteins from vascular space, consequent tissue swelling, and increased immune cell response.

When white cells arrive at the site of inflammation, they bring inflammatory LTs with 200 to 20,000 times the bronchoconstrictor action of histamine. These PGs and LTs are formed from dietary essential fatty acids, primarily from arachidonic acid, in a cascade of chemical reactions facilitated by cyclooxygenase enzymes. Miller (1996) affirmed that "the lipophilic [fat-loving] character of the constituents of essential oils must be regarded as the basis of their pharmacological activity. This property enables their small molecules to interact with the components of biological membranes. In this way they may influence the membrane permeability and the activity of the carriers, ionic channels, receptors, or membrane integrated enzymes, e.g. cyclooxygenase and lipoxygenase."

Numerous studies demonstrate that, like aspirin, essential oils diminish the inflammatory response to various noxious stimuli. The anti-inflammatory effects of German chamomile and lavender essential oils have been known and utilized for many years. Safayhi (1994) noted that *Chamomilla recutita* (German chamomile) is used in commercial preparations for treating inflammatory skin and bowel disease. In the process of distilling camomile EO, the compound matricine is transformed into chamazulene. Safayhi wanted to know whether matricine or chamazulene were responsible for inhibiting inflammatory LTs. He found that chamazulene, but not matricine, inhibited formation of LT B4, and blocked the peroxidation of arachidonic acid by cyclooxygenase and 12-lipoxygenase activity in human platelets. This indicates that the water or steam distilled EO of *Chamomilla recutita* is a more effective anti-inflammatory agent than the carbon dioxide extracted EO because the chamazulene is a transformation product formed in the heat of distillation. In 1996, Miller presented the results of his studies of three constituents of *Chamomilla recutita* on histamine release from rat peritoneal mast cells. Miller also found that chamazulene inhibited histamines in concentrations from 10^{-9} to 10^{-5} M, but stimulated release of histamine in concentrations above 10^{-5} M. By contrast, En-yne-dicyclo-ether had a moderate stimulation effect at concentrations lower than 10^{-4} M and a strong inhibiting effect higher concentrations. Miller found that chamazulene is not a strong inhibitor of histamine, but it does block the formation of LT B4. Safayhi confirmed this anti-inflammatory action of German chamomile, but not by the mechanism many people assumed.

Kim (1999) found that lavender EO inhibits immediate allergic reactions in mice and rats. He found that lavender EO inhibited histamine production and ear-swelling responses in rats stimulated by both topical and intradermal applications of a number of irritants. He used concentrations ranging from 1:500 to pure EO, and found that stronger concentrations inhibited the rats' ear-swelling more effectively. Kim also noted that lavender EO, in concentrations of 1:1000, 1:100, 1:10 and pure, had a significant inhibitory effect on anti-DNP IgE-induced tumor necrosis factor secretion from peritoneal mast cells. This shows that lavender has a number of benefits on the cellular level, as well as psychological effects.

A close acquaintance of mine provided a memorable personal case study. She developed facial hives of unknown etiology. She was already on oral prednisone for inflammatory bowel problems and asthma. The hives could be suppressed with higher doses of prednisone, but these higher doses left her feeling tired throughout the day, so she did not want to take them. I suggested a blend of essential oils including German chamomile and lavender in a cream for topical use on her hives, and she eagerly agreed. Initially she used the cream with beneficial results on hives already arisen; her itching subsided, and they disappeared faster. Then she began using the cream as a preventive medication on her whole face every morning. She was delighted to find that this suppressed the recurrence of her facial hives. Her internist was impressed with these results, but did not ask for further information.

For arthritic and borderline emphysema cases, Frankincense may produce some better results than NSAIDs. One monograph (1998) on *Boswellia serrata* (Indian Frankincense) reports that *Boswellia* inhibits human leukocyte elastase (HLE) which stimulates mucus secretion and may be involved in the pathogenesis of emphysema. By contrast, NSAIDs used for the same ailments may disrupt of glycosaminoglycan synthesis, degenerating cartilege and causing articular damage in arthritic conditions. The EO *Boswellia* prevented degradation of glycosaminoglycan compared to controls, whereas NSAIDs (ketoprophen) accelerated glycosaminoglycan degradation.

The recent public attention given to Neem oil is not undeserved, but users must pay attention to proper dosage. SaiRam (1997) worked with NIM-76, the steam distilled volatile fraction of cold pressed Neem seed oil. NIM-76 has high spermicidal activity, but not the abortificient effect of whole Neem oil. SaiRam studied changes in white cell and immuno-globulin response in rats pretreated for five days with either 120 mg/kg or 300 mg/kg i.p. While immune responses were improved for both groups, the 120 mg/kg group's PMNs showed enhanced yeast uptake and NBT reduction, but the 300 mg/kg group showed no significant difference from controls. This indicates that 300 mg/kg exceeded the optimal dose—too much of a good thing is not better. In further support of this, SaiRam showed there was no change in antibody levels in the lower dose and an actual decrease in antibody titers in the higher dose. So the effectiveness of essential oils is not always proportional to the doses used; this is a very important precaution for would-be self-prescribers.

Drs. Nagata, Kenner, and other contributors have discussed the effectiveness of bupleurum compounds in other chapters of this book. Studying the anti-inflammatory activity of *Bupleurum gibraltaricum* in rats, Ocete (1989) found that the EO showed dose-dependent anti-inflammatory activity comparable to that of indomethacin, but the oral dose needed to be about thirty times the peritoneal dose to obtain comparable results. His comparisons of the components of bupleurum revealed differences in potency of the components, but that not all its anti-inflammatory responses are dose dependent over time. Lorente (1989) examined the effects of the EO of *Bupleurum fruticosum* as well as its major constituents, alpha-pinene and beta-pinene, and a combination of the two pinenes. He too found the whole EO effective in a dose dependent manner, but that 40 mg/kg of beta-pinene was more effective than 80 mg/kg. Against carrageenan-induced inflammation, he found the whole EO more effective than either alpha-pinene or beta-pinene or alpha-pinene plus beta-pinene. This suggests that yet other constituents contribute to the anti-inflammatory response. Martin (1993) studied the anti-inflammatory effects of the EO of *Bupleurum fruticescens*. He found the whole EO more effective than its major constituent beta-caryophyllene, and the EO approximately equal to a combination of beta-caryophyllene and alpha-pinene. Martin's major constituents varied substantially from the two previous studies with bupleurum, demonstrating that EO constituents can vary widely from variety to variety, from year to year, from location to location. This is very important to remember when venturing generalizations about essential oils. In other words, these studies are very exciting indications of medical applications of essential oils, but readers should not jump to the conclusions that the essential oils in their local health-food stores will produce identical effects.

Analgesic Action of Essential Oils

While some essential oils excel at inhibiting painful swelling, hives, and arthritic conditions, other essential oils have morphine-like analgesic effects, reducing sensitivity to pain itself. Al-Zuhair (1996) studied the effects of cardamom *(Elettaria cardamomum)* EO, finding that doses ranging from 50 to 1600 mcg/kg produced drowsiness, staggering gait, and absence of pain reflex in mice. Foot swelling was induced by carrageenan and then countered with indomethacin (30 mg/kg) or 175 or 280 mcg/kg of EO. The indomethacin dose proved intermediate in effectiveness between the two EO doses. In his test of analgesia to para-benzoquinone induced writhing response, Al-Zuhair compared similarly increasing dosages of cardamom EO and aspirin; they showed similar dose-response curves. The EO was also tested on prepared rabbit intestine; gradually increasing doses of EO inhibited spontaneous movement in a dose-dependent manner. As aspirin has a number of contraindications and side effects, it is highly interesting that an essential oil of a common herb like that of cardamom can exhibit similar pain-reducing effects.

Lorenzetti (1991) studied the analgesic activities of Brazilian lemongrass *(Cymbopogon citratus)* in the form of tea, EO, and various chromatographic fractions of the EO. His gas and thin-layer chromatography determined that the major fraction with analgesic activity was myrcene; he confirmed this with mass spectrometry. The tea, EO, and especially its myrcene fraction, were effective against inflammation induced by carrageenan and PGE2. Then he tested the EO and myrcene against the writhing effects of acetic acid and iloprost. The dose response curves were similar. Myrcene was also tested in mice using a hot plate test, measuring reaction time for withdrawal. The myrcene enabled a non-significant prolongation of reaction time, but not near the prolongation enabled by administration of morphine. Lorenzetti's rat paw hyperalgesic testing suggested that lemongrass EO and myrcene have a direct peripheral-acting analgesic effect similar to opiates; this is further supported by the absence of antipyretic effects on fever induced by endotoxin in rabbits.

Aydin (1998) reported the effects of essential oils from several *Nepeta* species, particularly *Nepeta caesarea*, on mechanical and thermal discomfort in rats. Using rats' tail-flick and hot-water tail immersion tests, Aydin studied this EO, which produced marked sedation in test animals, and found that it reduced rats' tail flicks from mechanical but not thermal pain. He concluded that this EO acts on specific opioid subtype receptors, excluding mu-opioid receptors. The next year, Aydin (1999) reported on additional *Nepeta* species from other locations in Turkey. Again, he found that *Nepeta italica* (from only one of three locations) was able to inhibit the tail-flick response in mice but showed no effective analgesia in the hot water tail immersion test. So a variety of studies of animals suggests there is more than one mode of action for the anti-inflammatory and analgesic effects of essential oils and their constituents. What remains in question is not whether essential oils have analgesic effects, but the mechanisms by which they produce analgesia—it should be remembered that even the mechanisms of aspirin and other pain relievers were unknown until very recently. But incomplete knowledge of mechanisms is not necessarily a reason to avoid use of otherwise effective modalities.

It is significant that a considerable variety of essential oils exert anti-inflammatory and analgesic actions. Most of the essential oils cited above were selected for their prominence in the "folk medicines" of their respective regions. This suggests that if distillation equipment were more available, people could locally harvest and prepare their own essential oils cheaply and effectively for their own use.

(3) Effects of Essential Oils on Metabolism of Sugars and Fats

In addition to retarding bacterial/fungal growth and inhibiting swelling and pain, some essential oils have profound effects on the metabolism of sugars and cholesterol, which in turn are importantly linked to diabetes, obesity, and hardened arteries.

Al-Hader (1994) studied the effects of the EO of *Rosmarinus offinalis* on glucose and insulin levels in normal and diabetic rabbits. Previous work had demonstrated that rosemary EO has antispasmodic and tracheal smooth muscle relaxing effects; he attributed this smooth muscle relaxation to inhibition of cytosolic free calcium concentrations. (Other work demonstrated that elevated cytosolic free calcium concentration is a trigger for insulin release from beta-pancreatic cells.) Al-Hader subjected his rabbits to a glucose tolerance test (GTT) with serum glucose and insulin levels measured; one group took Rosemary EO before the glucose while the other group did not. The EO group showed higher glucose levels, with the differences from controls growing more significant from 60 to 90 to 120 minutes. The insulin level was lower at 30 minutes and not significantly different after that. Only after six hours did the diabetic rabbits receiving EO show significantly higher glucose levels. It appears that the hyperglycemic effect requires a normal pancreas to inhibit insulin release. So while rosemary will not dramatically affect a diabetic pancreas, it is an EO to keep in mind for helping hypoglycemic patients whose pancreas may over-release insulin in response to a glucose challenge.

Effects of Essential Oils on Lipid Metabolism

Yasni built upon his previous work showing that the EO of *Curcuma xanthorrhiza* (Javanese turmeric) lowered glucose activity in diabetic rats and lowered triglycerides in both normal and diabetic rats. In his 1994 study, he used turmeric EO and 10 hexane-soluble subfractions of turmeric EO to find its primary active constituents. (65 percent of the EO is alpha-curcumene.) He added EO (0.02 percent) to rat chow; this resulted in lower hepatic triglyceride concentration and stable serum triglyceride levels in two weeks time. When he added the hexane-soluble fraction (0.5 percent) to rat chow, it resulted in lower liver and serum triglyceride levels and higher concentrations of HDL in two weeks time. Examination of the rat livers after these trials revealed that both groups had lower hepatic fatty acid synthesis. In cultured rat hepatocytes, the hexane soluble fraction containing alpha-curcumene most suppressed the synthesis of fatty acids from [14C]acetate, demonstrating that alpha-curcumene is an active principle lowering triglycerides. Other subfractions also suppressed the synthesis of fatty acids from [14C]acetate in cultured rat hepatocytes, indicating that several constituents of turmeric lower liver and serum lipids. Yasni's study took only two weeks, and very low concentrations of turmeric EO, to effect changes in liver enzymes that affect the liver, and eventually serum triglycerides and cholesterol. Considering the tremendous sums that are already being invested in cholesterol-lowering foods and medications, it would be fascinating to see longer trials done testing the effects of oil of turmeric on human cholesterol!

Elson (1989) studied the impact of 140 mg of lemongrass EO daily on the serum cholesterol of 22 hypercholesterolemic patients for 90 days. The patients were selected because they had each undergone coronary bypass heart surgery within the previous seven years and had a serum cholesterol of over 250 mg/dl despite a diet strictly limited in fat, calories, and cholesterol intakes. The group as a whole showed a decreased average cholesterol ($p<0.06$), but the investigators noticed that the results fell into a bimodal distribution. Eight subjects responded well to the trial and fourteen were resistant. The responders tended to have higher starting triglycerides, a higher body mass index and required 20 percent fewer calories to maintain body weight. So for some people with elevated serum lipids, something as simple as 140 mg of lemongrass EO a day can make a significant difference in lowering cholesterol levels. After the lemongrass supplement was discontinued, by 90 days, the eight reduced-cholesterol patients returned to pre-study levels. This post-study evaluation shows that lemongrass EO was an active principle in lowering serum cholesterol in the responder group, but does not reveal the mechanism of action.

Nikolaevskii (1990) studied the essential oils of lavender, monarda, and basil on the course of experimental atherosclerosis in rabbits. Inhalation of lavender and monarda in concentrations of 0.1-2 mg/m^3 produced no change in serum cholesterol, but did diminish cholesterol in the aorta and reduce "atherosclerotic plaques" in the aorta. This decrease in cholesterol in the aorta following inhalation of lavender and monarda, especially with no change in serum cholesterol, recalls some theories that bacterial infection or inflammation are part of the process of atherosclerosis. Without further research we cannot jump to conclusions, but these thoughts may prompt new research.

While such scientific research is still in its infancy, the relative availability, ease of administration, low danger of side-effects, and cost-efficiency of essential oils to reduce cholesterol is another exciting prospect for the practice of holistic and complementary medicine.

Standards

The above listing of studies poses some exciting prospects for the application of essential oils. Unfortunately, as we have repeatedly noted, it is not sufficient simply to buy a bottle of essential oils and begin self-healing. Among the most serious problems is the establishment and maintenance of standards of purity of the essential oils available on the market. The most important standards concern the purity of the essential oils and truth in labeling the essential oils.

Some people and companies mislabel contents of EO bottles. For example, birch and wintergreen oils contain high percentages of methyl salicylate; sometimes pure chemical methyl salicylate is sold as if it were one of these oils. There is no warning that methyl salicylate can be toxic either in repeated small dosages or in one large dose (Lee, 1997); nor is there any warning that people sensitive to aspirin should avoid this product.

There is often no warning that most essential oils must be diluted. Some people and companies in the USA tell people to use these essential oils neat (undiluted) on the skin. Truth in labeling is important because if someone dilutes an oil, for example, oregano, and tells people it is pure, the unsuspecting person who buys the diluted oil first overpays, often dearly, for the product, and second, comes to think it is safe to use in high concentrations. The next time she buys a pure oregano oil and uses it in the dilutions she used with her previous purchase, the EO will irritate the skin. She will believe the second oil is defective! Recently, a woman phoned Aroma Medica™ looking for two essential oils. We told her that we did not sell them because manufacturers rarely label them accurately, and because people tend to misuse them. We told her that they always must be diluted in carrier oils because they can be strong skin irritants. She responded, "Oh, is that why I have a red, burning mark on my face where I put some just a while ago?"

We have already alluded to a number of ways that essential oils are adulterated. All of those present a deviation from good ethical practice, especially since users can be physically injured by the substitution. If not injured physically, the person is injured financially, because they have overpaid for a lesser product.

Another standard that is important has to do with the packaging of pure essential oils. For retail purposes, essential oils should come in small glass bottles with orifice reducers. The glass is inert and will protect the oils. Many oils interact chemically with plastic, dissolving molecules of plastic into the EO, or even weakening the plastic container. In addition, plastic is porous, so that oxidation of the EO can occur even in a closed plastic container. The orifice reducer serves two purposes; it enables the user to measure by counting drops of oil, and it makes accidental poisoning less likely by preventing children from inadvertently drinking a whole bottle of EO.

Education Desired

The next issue of safety is a thorough knowledge of and respect for the essential oils. As stated previously, essential oils are the most powerful concentration of active botanical constituents that we have. People using or recommending essential oils need to know what they are doing. This leads directly into our next section on education.

To use essential oils one needs to appreciate that very tiny doses suffice to bring about a shift toward healing in the body. As reiterated above, more is not always better when using essential oils. When using a holistic approach to healing, using the least force or influence to stimulate the body's own healing mechanisms, generally only very tiny quantities of essential oils are used or needed at any one time. If one is using them by inhalation, it takes only a few molecules to stimulate olfactory sensations. These olfactory sensations go directly from the olfactory nerve to major control centers in the brain, to the limbic system, thalamus, hypothalamus and then to the cortex and the rest of the body. Years ago, John Steele studied EEG changes evoked by smelling essential oils. The changes were almost instantaneous (personal communication). I have recommended inhalation of some essential oils such as frankincense or sandalwood to slow and deepen respiration, for meditation, and for quelling anxiety. I have used inhalation of other essential oils to stimulate a somnolent audience. Once, confronted with a sleepy audience late at night, I asked them to compare two varieties of basil by sniffing their essential oils. I was really using mentally stimulating essential oils so we could have an interesting discussion. It worked beautifully; the audience came alive!

There are many "first-aid" uses for essential oils that general populations can learn, just as they learn any OTC healing remedies. As more remedies and supplements are available, more education of the general public is necessary. Recently, I wrote an article entitled "Lavender Essential Oil: First Aid Kit in a Bottle" for an alternative/complementary newsletter, describing the uses of lavender EO and the advantages of keeping a small bottle handy at home. One memorable account concerned a woman who burned her hand terribly while removing sticky buns from her oven. First, the caramelized goo overran the pan and burned her; she withdrew her hand, dropped the potholder, then grabbed the pan with her bare hand. Her hand was intensely red and painfully burned. She ran her burned hand under cold water, then placed it in a bowl with water and ice. Then she gently dabbed some lavender

EO on the burned areas of her hand. Over the next forty minutes, the people present watched her hand return to its normal color, witnessed her move all her fingers, and heard her say that it no longer hurt. Those unfamiliar with lavender EO were absolutely incredulous. I saw another burn of similar magnitude, not treated in this way, require an emergency room visit, topical antibiotics, extensive dressings, and several visits to a plastic surgeon, leaving an unhappy woman who could not use her hand for six weeks.

Believing in the benefits of aromatherapy, I founded the Aroma Medica™ line of healing products that combine diluted essential oils for safety. Like other OTC remedies, these products require no knowledge of chemistry or even of essential oils. To benefit from such premixed products, a patient need only know when, how, and how much to use. Continuing research in essential oils' safety and stability will further increase the market for such OTC products.

When professional diagnosis and treatment are required, patients need practitioners with a systematic scientific understanding of health and physiology. Aromatherapy professionals need to understand the actions of the essential oils, including how they help a person return to healthy balance. With a solid background, medical practitioners can diagnose and treat patients by incorporating essential oils with other modalities. For example, a patient may benefit greatly from aromatherapy massage as an integral part of a total care program for arthritis, cancer, depression, anxiety or high blood pressure. Practitioners must understand the safety issues in using essential oils and must clearly communicate to patients how to best use the essential oils they prescribe. Practitioners must also understand how their EO prescriptions may complement, interact with, or counteract other treatments their patients receive from other health care professionals.

There are no governmental licensing or certification programs for aromatherapists in the English-speaking world today. For someone to practice aromatherapy currently, they need credentials in another medical modality such as allopathic medicine, nursing, massage, chiropractic, or naturopathy, that does license professionals. Their practice is legally limited by the licenses they hold, and morally limited by their knowledge and experience. (An exception might be healers working in traditional cultures, following many years of disciplined apprenticeship through which they learn traditionally safe as well as effective practices.) Many aromatherapists in the USA, Canada, Australia, and Great Britain are working to establish educational standards for aromatherapy. Introductory educational programs might train people to use a few essential oils safely for first aid like other OTC remedies, and convey elementary knowledge about the physiological effects of the essential oils on the body. More advanced educational programs should cover in-depth education in all related subjects, including a wider range of essential oils as well as introductory EO chemistry. We may hope that the popularity, safety, and cost-effectiveness of EO treatments will extend the present use of essential oils for health maintenance, and lead to professional organizations and standards like those in allopathic medicine, dentistry, or nursing.

Cost-Effectiveness

Aromatherapy can be a very cost-effective modality, either standing alone for first aid, or integrated into a larger health care program. Many of the "workhorse" essential oils most commonly used for healing purposes are inexpensive compared to pharmaceutical alternatives. The "perfumey" floral essential oils tend to be expensive, but often a tiny amount is effective, or a less expensive alternative will suffice as a substitute.

On August 30, 1999, in the *Wall Street Journal*'s article, "Americans to Spend More on Prescription Drugs," the National Association of Chain Drug Stores estimated that consumers would spend $121.6 billion on prescription drugs alone that year—an average of more than a dollar a day, every day, for every single person in the country. This continues the trend of more costly prescriptions, even though a growing number of former prescription drugs are becoming available over-the-counter. (Of course, the vast majority of Americans are not on daily prescriptions, so the daily cost per user is in fact many times higher.) This cost for medical care does not include visits to doctors, laboratory studies, diagnostic procedures, imaging studies, treatments, hospitalizations, surgeries, nor administrative charges and profits for insurance companies. Like many other complementary/integrated modalities, aromatherapy is low-tech. It involves listening to and talking with patients, touching them, encouraging them to be aware of their sensations, asking them to participate in their own care and well-being...literally asking people to stop to smell the flowers. In our increasingly busy and impersonal world, aromatherapy can be a fragrant respite indeed, that benefits all those using essential oils.

I deeply hope that aromatherapy and other complementary/integrated modalities like those represented in this book will change the way people take care of themselves in the years to come. I look forward to the day when our ancestors'—and primal peoples'—remedies will come full-circle to find a natural and beneficial place in our lives again.

References

al-Hader, A.A., Hasan, Z.A., Aqel, M.B. (1994). "Hyperglycemic and insulin release inhibitory effects of Rosmarinus officinalis." *Journal of Ethnopharmacology*, 43(3), 217–21.

al-Zuhair, H. et al., (1996). "Pharmacological studies of cardamom oil in animals." *Pharmacological Research*, 34(1–2), 79–82.

Aydin, S., Beis, R., Ozturk, Y., et al; (1998). "Nepetalactone: A new opioid analgesic from Nepeta caesarea Boiss." *Journal of Pharmacy and Pharmacology*, 50(7), 813–7.

Aydin, S., et al. (1999) "Analgesic activity of Nepeta italica L." *Phytotherapy Research*, 13(1), 20–3.

Brandao, M.G.L., Freire, N., Vianna-Soares, C.D. (1998). "Surveillance of phytothera-peutic drugs in the state of Minas Gerais: Quality assessment of commercial samples of chamomile." *Cad Saude Publica*, 14(3), 613–6.

Buck, D.S., Nidorf, D.M., Addino, J.G. (1994). "Comparison of two topical preparations for the treatment of onychomycosis: Melaleuca alternifolia (tea tree) oil and clotrimazole." *Journal of Family Practice*, 38(6): 601–5.

Caccioni, D.R., Guizzardi, M., Biondi, D.M., et al. (1998). "Relationship between volatile components of citrus fruit essential oils and antimicrobial action on Penicillium digitatum and Penicillium italicum." *International Journal of Food Microbiology*, 43(1–2), 73–9.

Carson, C.F., Cookson, B.D., Farrelly, H.D., et al. (1995). "Susceptibility of methicillin-resistant Staphylococcus aureus to the essential oil of Melaleuca alternifolia." *Journal of Antimicrobial Chemotherapy*, 35(3): 421–4.

Carson, C.F., Riley, T.V. (1995). "Antimicrobial activity of the major components of the essential oil of Melaleuca alternifolia." *Journal of Applied Bacteriology*, 78(3), 264–9.

Chinou, I.B., Roussis, V., Perdetzoglou, D., et al. (1996). "Chemical and biological studies on two Helichrysum species of Greek origin." *Planta Medica*, 62(4), 377–9.

Cox, S.D., et al. (1998). "Tea tree oil causes K+ leakage and inhibits respiration in Escherichia coli." *Letters of Applied Microbiology*, 26(5), 355–8.

Demetzos, C., Stahl, B., Anastassaki, T., et al. (1999). "Chemical analysis and antimicrobial activity of the resin Ladano, of its essential oil and of the isolated compounds." *Planta Medica*, 65(1), 76–8.

Elson, C. E., Underbakke, G. L., Hanson, P., et al. (1989). "Impact of lemongrass oil, an essential oil, on serum cholesterol." *Lipids*, 24(8), 677–9.

Gustafson, J.E., Liew, Y.C., Chew, S., et al. (1998). "Effects of tea tree oil on Escherichia coli." *Letters of Applied Microbiology*,1998, March; 26(3): 194–8.

Hammer, K.A., Carson, C.F., Riley, T.V., (1999). "Influence of organic matter, cations and surfactants on the antimicrobial activity of Melaleuca alternifolia (tea tree) oil in vitro." *Journal of Applied Microbiology*, 86(3), 446–52.

Jacobs, M.R., Hornfeldt, C.S., (1994). "Melaleuca oil poisoning." *Journal of Clinical Toxicology*, 32(4), 461–4.

Kim, H.M., Cho, S.H. (1999). "Lavender oil inhibits immediate-type allergic reaction in mice and rats." *Journal of Pharmacy and Pharmacology*, 51(2), 221–6.

Lachowicz, K.J., Jones, G.P., Briggs, D.R., et al. (1998). "The synergistic preservative effects of the essential oils of sweet basil (Ocimum basilicum L.) against acid-tolerant food microflora." *Letters in Applied Microbiology*, 26(3), 209–14.

Lee, K.K., Chan, T.Y., Lee C.W. (1997). "Improvements are needed in the existing packaging of medicated oils containing methyl salicylate." *Journal of Clinical Pharmacology and Therapeutics*, 22(4), 279–81.

Lima, E.O., Gompertz, O.F., Giesbrecht A.M., et al.. (1993). "In vitro antifungal activity of essential oils obtained from offifinal plants against dermatophytes." *Mycoses*, 36(9–10), 333–6.

Lorente, I., Ocete, M.A., Zarzuelo, A., et al. (1989). "Bioactivity of the essential oil of Bupleurum fruticosum." *Journal of Natural Products*, 52(2), 267–72.

Lorenzetti, B.B., Souza, G.E., Sarti, S.J. et al. (1991). "Myrcene mimics the peripheral analgesic activity of lemongrass tea." *Journal of Ethnopharmacology*, 34(1), 43–8.

Mahmoud, A.-L.E. (1994). "Antifungal action and antiaflatoxigenic properties of some essential oil constituents." *Letters in Applied Microbiology*, 9(19),110–113.

Mangena, T., Muyima, N.Y. (1999). "Comparative evaluation of the antimicrobial activities of essential oils of Artemisia afra, Pteronia incana and Rosmarinus officinalis on selected bacteria and yeast strains." *Letters in Applied Microbiology*, 28(4), 291–6.

Martin, S., Padilla, E., Ocete, M.A., et al. (1993). "Anti-inflammatory activity of the essential oil of Bupleurum fruticescens." *Planta Medica*,59(1), 533–36.

Maudsley, F., Kerr, K.G. (1999). "Microbiological safety of essential oils used in complementary therapies and the activity of these compounds against bacterial and fungal pathogens." *Supportive Care Cancer*, 7(2),100–2.

Miller, T., Wittstock, U., Lindequist, U., Teuscher, E. (1996). "Effects of some components of the essential oil of chamomile, *Chamomilla recutita*,on histamine release from rat mast cells." *Planta Medica*, 62(1), 60–1.

Mishra, A.K., Dubey, N.K. (1994). "Evaluation of some essential oils for their toxicity against fungi causing deterioration of stored food commodities." *Applied Environmental Microbiology*, 60(4), 1101–5.

Nenoff, P., Haustein, U.F., Brandt, W. (1996). "Antifungal activity of the essential oil of Melaleuca alternifolia (tea tree oil) against pathogenic fungi in vitro." *Skin Pharmacology*, 9(6), 388–94.

Nikolaevskii,V.V., Kononova, N.S., Pertsovskii, A.I., Shinkarchuk, I.F. (1990). "Effect of essential oils on the course of experimental atherosclerosis." *Patol ogicheskaia Fiziol Eksp Ter*, 34 (5), 52–3.

Ocete, M.A., Risco, S., Zarzuelo, A., Jimenez, J. (1989). "Pharmacological activity of the essential oil of Bupleurum gibraltaricum: Anti-inflammatory activity and effects on isolated rat uteri." *Journal of Ethnopharmacology*, 25(3), 305–13.

Ouattara, B., Simard, R.E., Holley, R.A., et al. (1997). "Antibacterial activity of selected fatty acids and essential oils against six meat spoilage organisms." *International Journal of Food Microbiology*, 37(2–3), 155–62.

Pattnaik, S., Rath, C., Subramanyam, V.R. (1995). "Characterization of resistance to essential oils in a strain of Pseudomonas aeruginosa(VR–6)." *Microbios*, 81(326), 29–31.

Pattnaik, S., Subramanyam, V.R. (1996). "Antibacterial and antifungal activity of ten essential oils in vitro." *Microbios*, 86(349), 237–46.

Pattnaik, S. Subramanyam, V.R., Bapaji, M. et al. (1997). "Antibacterial and antifungal activity of aromatic constituents of essential oils." *Microbios*, 89(358), 39–46.

Ross, S.A., el-Keltawi, N.E., Megella, S.E. (1980). "Antimicrobial activity of some Egyptian aromatic plants." *Fitotherapia*, 51, 201–205.

Safayhi, H., Sabieraj J., Sailer, E., et al. (1994). "Chamazulene: An antioxidant-type inhibitor of leukotriene B4 formation." *Planta Medica*, 60, 410–13.

SaiRam M., Sharma, SK., Ilavazhagan, G., et al. (1997). "Immunomodulatory effects of NIM-76.-a volatile fraction from Neem oil." *Journal of Ethnopharmacology*, 55(2), 133–9.

Schaller, M., Korting, H.C. (1995). "Allergic airborne contact dermatitis from essential oils used in aromatherapy." *Clinical and Experimental Dermatology*, 20(2), 143–5.

Smith-Palmer, A., Stewart, J., Fyfe, L. (1998). "Antimicrobial properties of plant essential oils and essences against five important food-borne pathogens." *Letters of Applied Microbiology*, 26(2), 118–22.

Soderberg, T.A., et al. (1996). "Toxic effects of some conifer resin acids and tea tree oil on human epithelial and fibroblast cells." *Toxicology*, 22; 107(2), 99–109.

Suresh, B., Sriram, S., Dhanaraj S.A., et al. (1997). "Anticandidal activity of Santolina chamaecyparissus volatile oil." *Journal of Ethnopharmacology*, 55(2), 151–9.

Syed, T.A., Qureshi, Z.A., Ali, S.M. (1999). "Treatment of toenail onychomycosis with 2 percent butenafine and 5 percent Melaleuca alternifolia (tea tree) oil in cream." *Tropical Medicine and International Health*, 4(4), 284–7.

Takaisi-Kikuni, N.B., Kruger, D.Gnann, W., Wecke, J. (1996). "Microcalorimetric andelectron microscopic investigation on the effects of essential oil from Cymbopogon densiflorus on Staphylococcus aureus." *Microbios*, 88(354), 55–62.

Viollon, C., Chaumont, J.P. (1994). "Antifungal properties of essential oils and main components on Cryptococcus neoformans." *Mycopathologia*,128(3), 151–3.

Wan, J., Wilcock, A., Coventry, M.J. (1998). "The effect of essential oils of basil on the growth of Aeromonas hydrophila and Pseudomonas fluorescens." *Journal of Applied Microbiology*, 84(2), 152–8.

Yasni, S., Imaizumi, K., Sin, K., et al. (1994). "Identification of an active principle in essential oils and hexane-soluble fractions of Curcuma xanthorrhiza Roxb. showing triglyceride-lowering action in rats." *Food and Chemical Toxicology*, 32(3), 273–278.

Monograph. (1998) "Boswellia serrata." *Alternative Medical Review*, 3(4), 306–7.

7.

Holistic Aromatherapy in the U.S.
Uniting Body, Mind, and Spirit

Lizette C. Pirtle, C.A., M.A.
International Affiliations Coordinator, NAHA

Sylla Sheppard-Hanger, C.A.
Chair of Safety Committee, NAHA

Introduction

This chapter provides an inclusive definition of "Holistic Aromatherapy," considers the status of this practice in the United States, and reports on the challenges and the problems that aromatherapy faces. It presents scientific evidence supporting the effectiveness of essential oils, and reflects on the inherent problems with existing aromatherapy studies, while proposing considerations for future research. It also provides a comprehensive account of the current standards of safety, quality, consumer awareness, and education in the United States, and discusses the role of the National Association for Holistic Aromatherapy (NAHA) in these areas. It concludes with a review of the potential cost savings of holistic aromatherapy.

The Birth of Holistic Aromatherapy

Although aromatic plants have been used since the dawn of history,[1] modern aromatherapy is said to have commenced in 1937 with the publication of a book by French chemist René Gattefossé entitled *Aromathérapie: Les Huiles essentielles hormones végétales*.[2]

This book was one of the first attempts to begin a comprehensive and systematic study of the therapeutic uses of essential oils in recent times. During the same period, the French army surgeon Dr. Jean Valnet engaged in the study of the uses and properties of essential oils, leading to his publication of the aromatherapy classic *The Practice of Aromatherapy* in 1964.[3] Gattefossé used incomplete[4] (terpeneless) essential oils in many of his studies, but like Valnet, focused only on physical therapeutic effects.

Their contemporary, the biochemist Madame Marguerite Maury, introduced a holistic approach to the practice of aromatherapy by considering the spiritual and mental aspects of human existence in her methodology. She further proposed the need for "individual prescription," recognizing the important holistic postulate that individuals are inherently different. Madame Maury centered her practice on the application of highly diluted essential oils via the skin by massage or added to the bath, avoiding all other methods of administration.[5]

Although Mme. Maury proposed a holistic approach through her work, the stipulations of using essential oils exclusively through the skin and in low dilution restrict her practice of aromatherapy. In the United States, most practitioners incorporate other methods, using higher concentrations of essential oils when appropriate. They claim to follow a holistic approach, but because of the limiting associations of the term "holistic aromatherapy," they opt to use the single appellation "aromatherapy" to designate their profession. Unfortunately, the many definitions of the word "aromatherapy" lead to confusion and misconceptions.

The simplest definition of aromatherapy regards it as a healing modality based on aromas or aromatic substances, as set forth in Gattefossé's preface: "A therapy or cure using aroma, aromatics, scents."[6] The term "aromatherapy" itself contributes to the confusion, for it superficially implies a "smell-related" therapy, rather than the use of aromatics in many different healing applications. Uneducated consumers disregard the healing connotations of the word "therapy," understanding aromatherapy as the use of fragrant substances such as scented candles, potpourri, bath, and body products for purely aromatic purposes. A descriptive word is sometimes added in an effort to clarify the term, for example: cosmetic aromatherapy, clinical aromatherapy, medical aromatherapy, or holistic aromatherapy. In some cases such compound words elucidate the terminology, however they may add confusion at the consumer level.

Holistic Aromatherapy: The Whole Person—The Whole Essence—The Whole Practice

Existing definitions of aromatherapy concentrating only on certain methodologies fail to reflect the current and broader practice of this healing modality in the United States. We should redefine "Holistic Aromatherapy" as follows:

> Holistic Aromatherapy encompasses the inhalation, external and internal bodily as well as environmental applications of pure whole essential oils, hydrosols, or absolutes to restore or maintain physical, emotional, mental, as well as spiritual health and balance. It rests on the premise that "the whole is greater than the sum of the parts"; it treats the whole person in an attempt to unite body, mind, and spirit, recognizing that essential oils work on all three levels. It heeds individual differences while considering the interconnectedness among human beings and the environment. Its objective is to treat the causes of disease and not just the symptoms. Its focus is as strong on prevention as it is on treatment. Environmental applications effectively sanitize, disinfect, and deter insects naturally, without poisoning the environment.

The concepts included in this definition are not new; however, to accurately reflect the current practice of holistic aromatherapy in the United States, no methods of administration should be excluded. This comprehensive definition is also required in order to separate holistic aromatherapy from other methodologies and to avoid mistaken associations with trendy aromatic products that neither contain natural essential oils nor offer therapeutic value.

One of the differences between holistic aromatherapy and other methodologies is the consideration of the entire being. For instance, when relieving muscle pain or tension, a holistic aromatherapist may create a blend of essential oils to act upon the client emotionally and psycho-spiritually, as well as to relax the muscles and relieve pain. In choosing essential oils and carriers, the holistic practitioner attempts to address the underlying cause of the discomfort, considering the individual and the premise that the chosen oils act on all levels (body-mind-spirit). Conversely, non-holistic aromatherapists only treat muscle conditions; they are not necessarily concerned with the causes of the problem, much less its psychological or spiritual aspects. Holistic aromatherapists therefore need a thorough knowledge and comprehension of the effects of the therapy on the body and mind, including pharmacology, anatomy, physiology, pathology, psychology, and the body's energy system. Also required is a solid foundation on which practitioners can draw to connect with their clients to help them achieve harmony with themselves, their fellow human beings, their circumstances, and their psycho-physical environment.

A holistic aromatherapist uses the purest ingredients, specifically essential oils and hydrosols that are obtained with the least amount of human intervention, using only mechanical and physical forces during the extraction process. Adulteration either by the addition of natural or synthetic chemical substances or by the removal of certain constituents is not acceptable to a holistic aromatherapist. On the other hand, the non-holistic practitioner is not necessarily concerned with purity and quality.

Absolutes are oils that result from use of solvents to draw out essential oils from plant material. In the past, residue from these solvents was thought to interfere with the purity associated with holistic aromatherapy. In holistic practice, lack of purity is the most quoted explanation for the sparing use of absolutes; it leads some practitioners to avoid and others to decry absolutes. At present, many absolutes are virtually solvent-free, but the controversy surrounding their use remains. Despite disagreement among practitioners, absolutes are necessary to obtain essences from certain flowers and herbs that have very low yields or produce inferior oils with distillation. Moreover, the spiritual effects of some absolutes advise their inclusion in holistic aromatherapy. Christopher McMahon provides an excellent example of such subtle actions in his description of the spiritual effects of the Lotus absolute.[7]

Challenges Facing Holistic Aromatherapy in the US

Today, holistic aromatherapy faces many challenges, beginning with the very nature of its tools: essential oils are powerfully concentrated natural chemicals that can pose harm if used without safety and quality guidelines. The efficacy and safety of essential oils are directly related to their quality; thus the need for rigor in standards, diagnosis, and application. The dramatic spread of aromatherapy in the last few years has magnified the need for practitioner education and public awareness of safety issues. Nor has this popularity resulted in unilateral acceptance; some health professionals still question its effectiveness and refuse to take it seriously. Although the number of validated clinical studies is mushrooming, the acceptance of the practice still rests largely on anecdotal accounts, suggesting the need for more formal research with tighter methodology. Another major issue confronting aromatherapy today is the need for education at multiple levels, suited to varied audiences that each require different approaches and levels of information. These groups include the public, home users of essential oils, aromatherapy practitioners, and other health professionals wishing to incorporate essential oils into their practices.

Safety Concerns

Effective aromatherapy requires knowledge of contraindications and toxicity; safe dosages, proper dilutions, timing of use, and product quality. Because essential oils are very concentrated substances, practitioners and home users must overcome the general notion that "more is better." In holistic aromatherapy, the reverse is actually true; less is preferred. Proper dosages and dilutions are linked to safety and toxicity levels, which vary from oil to oil and according to methods of administration, conditions to be treated, and health, age, and tolerance of the person. Beginners in aromatherapy tend to utilize only a few essential oils too regularly, posing the risk of sensitization reactions.

Most people benefit from essential oils, but certain sensitive atopic patients—those who show reactions to common perfume or suffer from environmental allergies—may experience skin irritations or allergies from essential oils.[8] Children and elderly patients require much lower dosages than healthy adults, and may be too sensitive for the use of certain essential oils even at very low doses.

Certain oils are contraindicated by particular conditions. For example, camphor, oregano, and yarrow are contraindicated for asthma sufferers.[9] Juniper, parsley, and ravensara anisata should not be used by chronic kidney disease patients.[10] People with a history of epilepsy should avoid rosemary, lavender stoechas, and sage.[11] Cinnamon, clove, and rosemary should not be used by people prone to gastric ulcers.[12]

All essential oils should be used with caution during pregnancy. Except for those few proven safe, such as rose, neroli, lavender, and chamomile, the general recommendation is to completely avoid using oils during the first trimester.[13] Mugwort, parsley, pennyroyal, sage, sassafras, sage, tansy, thuja, rue, and wormwood are known to have abortifacient effects and so should never be used during pregnancy.[14]

Some essential oils can be irritants, such as allspice, ajowan, bay leaf, clove bud and leaf, cassia, chervil, cinnamon, horseradish, mustard, mints, and dwarf pine.[15] Some essential oils are known skin sensitizers causing allergic reactions and so are restricted by the International Fragrance Research Association (IFRA). These essential oils include aniseed, elecampane, calamus, cassia, cinnamon bark and leaf, citronella, costus root, fennel bitter, jasmine absolute, mimosa absolute, cpoponax, peru balsam, pines, spearmint, tolu balsam, turpentine, and styrax gum.[16] Citrus oils such as expressed bergamot, combava, lemon, lime, tangerine, mandarin, May Chang, bitter and sweet orange are phototoxic—they should not be used on the skin prior to sun exposure; other phototoxic oils include angelica root, lemon verbena, cumin, and rue.[17]

From a toxicological perspective, under appropriate and specified conditions of use, most common essential oils are relatively safe. Nonetheless, some essential oils should be used with caution and others completely avoided. Internal consumption of certain essential oils can be harmful, moderately or highly toxic, and so should be eschewed. Orally "harmful" oils include bitter almond, jaborandi, mugwort, santolina, sassafras, tansy, tonka bean, thuja, wormseed and wormwood; orally moderately toxic oils include high-chavicol basil, birch, rectified cade, camphor, deertongue, elecampane root, common mugwort, rue, turpentine, and wintergreen; orally highly toxic oils include boldo leaf, horseradish, mustard, and savin. In the absence of conclusive testing, we should consider such orally toxic oils unsuited to dermal application as well, for safety's sake.[18]

In addition to the dangers inherent in some essential oils and the possible complications of improper dosages, unscrupulous or uninformed companies produce "aromatherapy" products using synthetic fragrances, chemical extractors, or poor quality oils with no thought (or no knowledge!) of current safety practices. In America, the National Association for Holistic Aromatherapy (NAHA), a non-profit educational organization, has mandated committees to address these safety and quality concerns.[19] The goal of NAHA is self-regulation: to ensure that proper safety, quality, educational, and ethical standards are clearly defined, enforced, and consequently followed by the membership. (The role of NAHA in dealing with the challenges facing aromatherapy is discussed at length below.) Stringent standards imposed by an association such as NAHA are more desirable and effective in the practice of aromatherapy than government intervention or regulation.

Despite safety concerns, holistic aromatherapy has a proper and important place in assisting people to live healthier and more balanced lives. Essential oils offer immense psychological benefits, specifically in the reduction of stress. They can aid in resolving emotional imbalances as well as reducing the discomfort, anxiety, and pain related to many diseases. Further, essential oils can be very effective in dealing with certain pathogens, offering an alternative to synthetic antibiotics and other chemicals used for minor first aid.

Holistic aromatherapy is a complementary rather than an alternative practice, inappropriate as the sole treatment for many conditions. It should not be thought to treat life-threatening diseases, although under appropriate medical supervision, it may be useful to relieve symptoms and to assist patients in pain control, and in dealing with emotional and psycho-spiritual repercussions of their conditions.

Testing the Effectiveness of Holistic Aromatherapy

Scientific as well as anecdotal evidence corroborates that essential oils exhibit a myriad of therapeutic effects. The practice of aromatherapy is said to be most effective in treating minor acute infections, improving immune response, and achieving or maintaining emotional well-being through its stress-reducing calming effects.[20] Some essential oils work well to alleviate symptoms of respiratory ailments due to their expectorant,[21] antispasmodic,[22] and mucolytic[23] actions, while others have powerful vulnerary effects aiding in the healing of wounds and skin ulcers.[24]

Essential oils can be inhaled, applied topically, taken internally, and used in the environment for purposes of cleaning, sanitizing, or deterring insects; their methods of application determine how they will act on and eventually be eliminated from the body.[25]

Inhalation of essential oils can be accomplished by using steam,[26] micro-diffusers,[27] or by simply placing a few drops on a cotton ball or tissue and bringing it close to the nose. When inhaled, essential oil components entering the nasal passages stimulate the olfactory nerve and send electro-chemical messages directly to the limbic system of the brain. The limbic system is the seat of memory and learning as well as emotion; the inhalation of essential oils can stimulate and trigger changes in these centers.[28]

Ludvigson and Rottman (1989) used college students to test the effects of lavender and clove aromas on cognitive skills and affective reactions. They found that the scent of lavender negatively affected arithmetic reasoning (!) while the scent of cloves increased willingness and improved affective reactions to the test.[29] The messages created by the aromatic molecules and relayed through the limbic system are transmitted to the hypothalamus, the gland that acts as a regulator of hormonal imbalances and emotional states such as anxiety and depression.[30] Yamaguchi (1990) and Sugano (1992) showed that inhalation of aromas such as sandalwood, bergamot, chamomile,[31] rose, or lavender[32] induces a state of relaxation and decreases anxiety levels. Birchall (1990) recorded EEG patterns indicating that the odor of lavender produced a de-stressing effect in humans.[33] Sugano (1991) tested orange fragrance for its effects on work efficiency, finding improvement in reaction times and increased α-band brain activity suggesting mental relaxation.[34]

External applications of essential oils show analgesic,[35] antiseptic, anti-fungal, anti-inflammatory, antispasmodic, and other beneficial properties.[36] Combining inhalation with dermal applications amplifies the stress-reducing effects of aromatherapy; this major benefit is propelling this form of healing to its current level of popularity. Such synergistic value is found when cold or hot compresses are used to apply essential oils in cases of inflammation, spasms, or pain. In an aromatherapy massage, where the inhalation of essential oils is accompanied by the therapeutic effects of touch, the synergistic relationship between therapist and client produces a richly beneficial outcome on several levels.[37] Wilkinson (1995) reports the effects of ordinary massage as compared to aromatherapy massage on patients receiving palliative care for cancer. The findings included a statistically significant reduction in pain as well as in anxiety and depression using essential oils rather than ordinary massage oil![38] Likewise, Stevenson (1994) reports a reduction of anxiety levels and improved relaxation of postoperative cardiac patients in an intensive care unit following a foot massage using Neroli oil for 20 minutes.[39]

Medical doctors and qualified aromatherapists can treat systemic problems such as infections by prescribing essential oils for internal use (oral ingestion). Given correct dosages, safety precautions, and purity confirmation, this approach works well for indigestion, as well as for bacterial, viral, and fungal infections. However, the toxicity, contraindications, and overdose dangers of essential oils taken internally are risks that should limit internal use to qualified practitioners; ingestion should not be undertaken by novices.

Other applications include using essential oils to repel insects and as antiseptic or sanitizing agents on the environment. Researchers in India have found that peppermint oil (*Mentha piperita*) repels adult mosquitoes and kills their larvae. A team led by Musharrah Ansari of the Malaria Research Center and Padma Vasudevan of the Center for Rural Development and Technology in Delhi tested peppermint oil on the larvae of three mosquito species—*Aedes aegypti* (which carries dengue fever), *Anopheles stephensi* (malaria) and *Culex quinquefasciatus* (filariasis and West Nile virus) and found various degrees of effectiveness at different concentrations.[40] Dube et al (1989) found the oil of basil (*Ocimum basilicum*) effective against the *Aloophora* species.[41] Other examples supporting insect repelling efficacy of essential oils are found in the works of Ansari and Razadan (1995)[42] and Watanabe et al (1993)[43]. Ansari and Razadan reported almost complete protection against *Anopheles culicifacies* (related to malaria) and other *anopheles* species using citronella, lemongrass, and palmarosa. Watanabe et al studied some of the constituents of *Eucalyptus camaldulensis*, specifically eucamalol, concluding that it was more effective than the standard insect repellent DEET against *Aedes aegypti*.

Ever since 1887, when Chamberlain published a groundbreaking paper describing the action of essential oils against anthrax spores,[44] essential oil vapors have been known to inhibit microorganisms. In another classic experiment forty years ago, J.C. Maruzella et al. (1960) tested the vapors from 133 essential oils against the killer bacterias *Escherichia coli, Staphylococcus aureus, Bacillus subtilis* var. *alterrimus, Streptococcus fecalis, Salmonella typhosa,* and *Mycobacterium avium.* Interestingly, 28 of the 133 essential oils tested were ineffective, but among the 105 antibacterial vapors, white and red thyme, cassia, savory, cinnamon, oregano, and cherry laurel produced the most positive effects.[45]

Measuring the Effectiveness of Holistic Aromatherapy

Measuring the effectiveness of holistic aromatherapy is a challenging task, because holism does not lend itself to isolating different components in order to determine their individual contributions to the outcome.[46] Furthermore, it is virtually impossible to "quantify" emotional and psycho-spiritual effects of this therapy. Despite the inherent limitations of quantitative studies when dealing with holistic practices, scientific studies are necessary to gain more knowledge about essential oils. While much evidence supporting holistic aromatherapy is anecdotal, a growing body of clinical studies supports specific uses and actions of essential oils. Such clinical studies are beginning to bridge the gaps between allopathic medicine and aromatherapy; and when they follow correct methodology, they can lend credibility to aromatherapy.

While scientific research on the uses and effects of essential oils is increasing, it is imperative to expand and improve scientific methodology. The vast majority of essential oil research to date depends on test-tube and petri-dish experiments, as summarized in Dr. DePaula's excellent chapter; we need *in vivo* studies to complement these *in vitro* findings. Animal testing is the standard means to determine the toxicity levels of essential oils, as of other synthetic drugs and chemicals. Animal skin and metabolism differs from humans', and emotional benefits are even less measurable in animals than in humans. Surely rats' writhing and tail-flick pain-responses are inadequate measures of emotional (not to mention psycho-spiritual) effectiveness, but rats are most widely used in essential oils research.

Extremely high dosages and unlikely methods of administration such as injections are common practices with laboratory rats. (We are well aware of the debates about animal testing, and are in sympathy with the plea that cruel methods of testing should be avoided.) In fact, it should be possible to measure the effectiveness and toxicity of essential oils by inhalation and diluted application tests on rats, rather than by megadoses and direct injections. Without other grounds, results from such extreme types of animal studies should not deter the use of essential oils in the small dosages and techniques used in aromatherapy, but sometimes they do.[47] Most oils used in perfumery have been tested dermally on humans, yet many essential oils used in aromatherapy have not been systematically analyzed for dermal safety in humans. Some essential oils have only been tested for one administration method (e.g., oral toxicity, but not dermal effects), and these results have been indiscriminately extrapolated against other modes of use.[48]

Other common methodological problems include the lack of identification of the botanical sources of essential oils used in the studies, the omission of quality analyses, and the use of single synthetic constituents. A failure to confirm botanical sources produces inconclusive results by not considering the differences that species, varieties, and places of origin produce in chemical composition and pharmacological and energetic actions of essential oils. Quality analysis must be conducted to exclude adulterated essential oils, since the adulterants themselves may skew the results of the studies. Emphasis must be placed on using whole, pure, natural essential oils and not single synthetic constituents, because the effectiveness of aromatherapy depends not on single isolated ingredients but on the synergy of the countless organic components naturally present in the oils. Whole essential oils are preferable because minor constituents have been shown to significantly complement and in some cases change the effects of major components.[49] Holistic practitioners believe in the wisdom of nature.

Given careful methodology, clinical studies lead to our greater knowledge and comprehension of the workings of essential oils, confirming or delimiting anecdotal accounts. Data resulting from scientific laboratory studies strengthen the foundations of holistic aromatherapy. As long as the practitioners' focus remains on the patients' entire being, their study of the parts assists in grasping and comprehending the whole. Ideally, clinical studies would seek to understand the effectiveness of holistic aromatherapy and measure its actions on the body, emotions, and psyche.

Aromatherapy Education

Aromatherapy has a broader range than many other healing modalities; each application requires a different degree of knowledge and training. Different education is required for treating a burn or sterilizing a cut than for inhaling a fragrance, and still more sophisticated medical training is required for effective medical use of aromatherapy in treatment of asthma or panic attacks. NAHA—the National Association for Holistic Aromatherapy—recognizes the need for these echelons of knowledge and degrees of training and has commenced a structured approach to deal with these challenges.

NAHA's Role in Safety, Quality, and Public Awareness

In the United States, mass advertising equates aromatherapy with scented candles, aromatic baths, floral shampoos, shower gels, bath soaps, and countless fragrant goods labeled "aromatherapy products." Despite the misleading messages of some commercials, a growing number of consumers have discovered the broad uses of essential oils and their applications in healing the body, mind, and psyche. However, aromatherapy professionals and responsible essential oil providers face the challenge of educating the public about the differences between generic so-called "aromatherapy products" and the therapeutic effects and cautions concerning true essential oils.

As more consumers turn to aromatherapy as a source of healing, public education becomes an increasingly urgent matter. The issues of quality standards, the need for more knowledge about effectiveness and the qualifications of practitioners also become critical. Product labeling, safety guidelines, and "seals of approval" by an independent body of experts are desirable measures. Since 1998, NAHA has taken important steps to face these issues; the results of these efforts are starting to materialize in formal programs that effectively address safety, quality, public awareness and education.

NAHA's membership reveals an increasing trend towards home use of essential oils by non-practitioners in the United States. Approximately 70 percent of NAHA members fall into the category of "Friends of Aromatherapy" (anyone interested in essential oils) while "Professional" and "Donor" members (professional practitioners and manufacturers) form smaller percentages.[50] By contrast, there are twelve professional associations in the United Kingdom representing a total of approximately 5,000 professional aromatherapists.[51] In 1991, The Aromatherapy Organizations Council (AOC) was formed to unite these different groups to present a unified front to the British government for the sake of seeking recognition of aromatherapy as a complementary therapy.[52] Regardless of the differences in their industries and membership distribution, the U.S. and the U.K. face the same challenges of safety, quality, and public awareness. However, the greater the use of aromatherapy by non-professionals, the greater the need for education, guidelines, and standards at the consumer level.

As the popularity of aromatherapy increases, so do the number of essential oil suppliers, aromatherapy products, and therapists. Aromatherapy is threatened by suppliers and practitioners who disregard safety and quality issues for the sake of quick profits. Such opportunistic vendors can be found in any market showing such rapid growth. However, when their health is at stake, consumers must be protected from misguided commercial interests.

One common commercial practice designed to improve profit margins and superficially to standardize aromas from one crop to the next is the addition of synthetic or natural substances to essential oils. These additives alter the chemical composition of essential oils, not only reducing their effectiveness, but inviting allergic reactions not to the oils but to the synthetic additives themselves. Thus, in aromatherapy, the safety and quality of essential oils are inherently linked. Quality is often reflected in higher prices, so consumers shopping for bargains are in danger of buying diluted or chemically altered oils.

A bigger challenge faced by aromatherapy is that essential oils, hydrosols, and vegetable oil carriers do not have to be adulterated to be inferior. Their quality is influenced by many factors such as: the health and chemical variety of the plant (chemotypes), variations in environmental growing conditions, production techniques, time of and care exercised during harvesting, methods of distillation or extraction, age and storage conditions.[53] These elements affect efficacy, and in many cases, the very safety of essential oils and aromatherapy products.

A good example of these differences is found in thyme (*Thymus vulgaris*), which has more than fifty varieties in the Mediterranean region alone. In southern France, at high altitudes, thyme is rich in the alcohols linalol and geraniol, its chemotype denominated by *Thymus vulgaris linalol*. This alcohol exhibits antiseptic, bactericidal, disinfectant, and antiviral actions with little toxicity. However, in the coastal areas of France near Saint-Tropez, a similar thyme is rich in the phenols carvacrol and thymol.[54] Phenols are also powerful antiseptic, bactericidal disinfectants, but may be toxic to the liver if taken orally, and may irritate the skin if applied dermally or the mucous membranes if inhaled. While some actions of these two chemical varieties of thyme are similar, their chemical differences can clearly lead to undesirable results if their origins and varieties are not clearly identified or if the users do not understand the differences. Therefore, full disclosure of origins, botanical varieties, and consequent precautions concerning essential oils are critical to ensure proper and safe usage.

In addition to stating the correct botanical sources of all ingredients, aromatherapy products diluted in vegetable oils or other carriers should carefully state the percentage dilution. If other chemical substances are added to—or originally present constituents have been removed from—a whole essential oil, these too should be disclosed on the label, in order that practitioners may take into account these changes in their uses of the oils.

To inform consumers, proper labeling of all essential oils and aromatherapy products is urgent. At a minimum, appropriate labeling includes English name, Latin binomial, chemotype (if several varieties exist), country/region of origin, extraction method, and date of production. Safe dosages, contraindications, and toxicity levels should be clearly displayed on each product. Unfortunately, the US Food and Drug Administration (FDA) prohibits some "guidelines for use" that could be interpreted to be therapeutic claims, but sources of this information can be listed or otherwise made available to consumers.

During the last few years, NAHA has taken significant measures to respond to these areas of concern. Members of NAHA's safety committee keep abreast of the latest research, disseminating their findings in a regular column of the Association's quarterly, *Aromatherapy Journal* (previously called *Scentsitivity*). In an effort to increase public awareness, this journal is now also being offered to bookstores around the country. Further efforts in public awareness include a toll-free telephone line and an informational website addressing consumers' personal questions about aromatherapy. NAHA frequently receives questions about the safe use of essential oils; these questions are forwarded to the safety committee for research and answers. The regional directors and other administrative members of NAHA also hold regular meetings open to the public in which safety of essential oils is a main topic of discussion.

To address quality issues, NAHA organized its TAP (True Aromatherapy Products) committee to develop a definition that would practically and legally ensure therapeutic quality and effectiveness, and to disseminate this information to the public. The TAP committee set out to answer the questions:

- What is "True Aromatherapy?"—a NAHA definition to include professional, practical and legal usage.
- What should constitute a "True Aromatherapy" product? (How could NAHA assay the purity and assure the authenticity of essential oils and "True Aromatherapy" products?)
- Should NAHA adopt a "Seal of Approval" for "True Aromatherapy" products? (What would be the concerns and liability of NAHA in the case of misuse of a "True Aromatherapy" product carrying the NAHA TAP seal?)
- How should NAHA communicate TAP information to the general public?

Much work has been done to answer these questions in the last two years. After an exhaustive analysis by the U.S. Government, the TAP seal was approved in March of 2000 through the Patents and Trademarks Office. The seal must pass through several Federal legal departments determining the criteria for its commercial use, so NAHA did not see its introduction until later.[55]

The approval of the NAHA TAP seal is a great victory for NAHA and for aromatherapy in the United States. Yet there is still much to be done in the area of quality assurance, such as the finalization of TAP criteria, legal adoption of marks and symbols, and meeting GC/MS requirements.

Once the seal is adopted, public education and awareness will become the major endeavor. In anticipation of this, NAHA formed a Public Awareness Campaign Advisory Panel to enlighten and inform the public about the health and wellness benefits of True Aromatherapy and True Aromatherapy Products. The panel recognizes that manufacturers, retailers, and educators in particular bring unique perspectives to the TAP process with their business and technical expertise and day-to-day interaction with the consumers of aromatherapy goods and services. So NAHA's public awareness campaign targets manufacturers, retailers, and educators, reinforced with an ongoing print and electronic media information campaign for the general public.[56]

NAHA'S Role in Developing Educational Standards

As previously discussed, aromatherapy education in the United States has two main concerns: home users and practitioners. The effort to formally educate non-practitioners is a novel and needed enterprise for all natural medicine therapies. As consumers take more responsibility for their own health, they are gravitating to natural therapies for maintenance and treatment. However, as this paper has exposed, natural does not always equate to harmless. Thus, when consumers make the choice to self-medicate with natural remedies, they create a need for education beyond marketing pamphlets, informational brochures and magazine articles.

Likewise the educational standards of those wishing to "treat" or "heal" others using natural therapies such as aromatherapy must be strict and clearly delineated.

In February, 2000, NAHA published a core curriculum required for the training of home users and aromatherapy professionals in its Directory of Schools and Educators. NAHA's Council for Aromatherapy Schools and Educators consists of members who adhere to NAHA standards of education. Members of the council have endorsed core curricula for two levels of education: home users and professional aromatherapy practitioners.

Educating Aromatherapy Home Users

NAHA's core curriculum consists of a minimum of 30 hours of training for home users wishing to use essential oils for themselves, their families and friends. A final examination requires that students demonstrate knowledge of actions, uses, and contraindications of the essential oils covered in the course, appropriate methods and dilutions for specific applications, as well as common ailments helped by these oils. Three case studies are also required, with the aim of teaching students a holistic approach to creating their blends. The course covers the following topics.[57]

- An introduction to the history of aromatherapy, focusing on ancient and traditional cultures
- The profiles of 12–20 essential oils. [The required oils are: *Cananga odorata* (Ylang-Ylang), *Chamaemelum nobile* (Roman Chamomile), *Citrus limon* (Lemon), *Citrus sinensis* (Sweet Orange), *Eucalyptus globulus* (Eucalyptus), *Lavandula angustifolia* (Lavender), *Melaleuca alternifolia* (Tea Tree), *Mentha X piperita* (Peppermint), *Pelargonium graveolens* (Geranium), *Rosa damascena* (Rose), *Rosmarinus officinale* (Rosemary), and *Salvia sclarea* (Clary Sage). Eight other essential oils are to be chosen by the school or instructor.]

- Production techniques and the quality of essential oils
- A basic knowledge of physiology: methods of absorption, general overview of the limbic, lymphatic, immune, and dermal systems
- The ways essential oils interact on physical and emotional levels
- A basic knowledge of aroma chemistry with contraindications and toxicity of essential oils
- The principles used in blending oils; different carriers and methods of application

Upon satisfactory completion of all requirements, a certificate of completion is awarded, with the understanding that it is not a license to practice aromatherapy except on self, family, and friends. This course is a prerequisite for the professional level course.

This is a commendable effort by NAHA to address the importance of formal education for safe home use of essential oils. Requiring schools to emphasize to students that this course does not provide them with enough knowledge to practice aromatherapy as a profession builds awareness of educational requirements and of safety concerns around essential oils usage. However, a clearer definition of the uses of essential oils that this level of education empowers the student to apply is in order. Additionally there is a need to specify which conditions may require the expertise of a qualified practitioner or physician and when the use of essential oils may be completely contraindicated without medical consultation. This information should be included in the Directory of Schools and Educators listing the core curriculum and sent to prospective students searching for reputable aromatherapy education providers. It is safe to assume that the growth of the Council will result in better and more information to the public, which could include these recommendations.

Educating Aromatherapy Practitioners

Currently, there is no government regulation of the professional practice of aromatherapy in the United States. In February, 2000, NAHA issued its first educational guidelines for the training of aromatherapy practitioners. The publication of the core curricula and the formation of the Council for Aromatherapy Schools and Educators are initial steps in a long process.

The NAHA core curriculum for Professional Aromatherapy Studies provides that schools offer a minimum of 200 hours of training and practical instruction focused on two areas: (1) Aromatherapy—Essential Oils Studies and (2) Anatomy and Physiology. Currently, there are no minimum hourly requirements for specific topics within the curriculum. However, "the future job of the Council is to create learning objectives, the content and level of knowledge required of students for each module."[58] The core curriculum for aromatherapy studies modules includes:

- History and development of aromatherapy
- Botanical taxonomy
- The properties of essential oils within holistic and clinical frameworks
- Methods of extraction
- Organic chemistry
- Carrier oils
- Blending techniques
- Methods of application
- Safety issues
- Consultation and treatment program design
- The basis of business development
- Legal and ethical issues

The core curriculum for Anatomy and Physiology modules includes:

- A knowledge of the structures and functions of the reproductive, circulatory, nervous, endocrine, lymphatic, immune, urinary and musculoskeletal systems
- In depth study of respiratory and integumentary (dermal/membrane) systems and the olfactory process
- Methods of application of essential oils to each system above, effects of essential oils on each of the above systems, and understanding a minimum of five (5) common ailments of each system that can be treated with the use of aromatherapy

People already holding degrees in health-related fields may waive the first of the Anatomy and Physiology requirements by demonstrating competence by examination; but the second and third requirements (not widely taught outside of aromatherapy circles) cannot be waived.

The school may grant an aromatherapy certificate to students who successfully complete the above course, pass examinations on every subject included in the course, and complete a research paper and a minimum of ten case histories. These certificates do not constitute a license or certification by NAHA itself; rather NAHA's guidelines serve as a third-party certification of the quality of the curriculum that the school offers to students. (NAHA had contemplated establishing a national certification examination, but after much consideration, NAHA recently decided to relinquish this project to America's Aromatherapy Registration Council with which NAHA works very closely.)

The Aromatherapy Registration Council and Educational Standards in Aromatherapy

In 1997, the Aromatherapy Registration Council (ARC), a non-profit Public Benefit Corporation, was established to serve as a registration board for aromatherapists. Although not directly affiliated with NAHA or any other group, the ARC has the complete support of NAHA. The ARC's Steering Committee for Educational Standards in Aromatherapy was formed in 1997 with the objective of establishing educational standards for the aromatherapy community. Since 1997, this ARC Steering Committee has been working with NAHA to define the roles of each organization. From its inception, the Committee considered a registration examination to ensure compliance with educational and ethical standards and other professional requirements. Graduates of aromatherapy courses wishing to become "registered practitioners" would be required to sit for a Board Exam, analogous to professional exams in law or real estate. This exam would cover the kind of core curriculum recently released by NAHA. For the past three years, members of the Steering Committee have compiled exams given at most aromatherapy schools; from that body of material they are creating the ARC exam, which they hope to become the standard for competency in the field. Grading guidelines for national standards are also being developed, and a code of ethics is being finalized. Graduates successfully completing the Board Exam will be issued practicing certificates and will be required to comply with the Code of Professional Ethics.[59]

Recommendations

As NAHA's Council of Aromatherapy Schools and Educators further defines its training objectives, it confronts students' vastly different levels of knowledge and expertise. It is critical that practitioners be taught to recognize the limitations both of aromatherapy itself and of their personal knowledge, and to know when to turn to other healing modalities, including allopathic medicine.

NAHA's objective of public protection also requires the protection of prospective aromatherapy students. Aromatherapy schools should be required to disclose information to assist students in making educated decisions when pursuing aromatherapy as a career choice. Schools and educators must be required to inform students about the limitations of the course; i.e., what the course will enable them to do and what it will not. Uninformed students can easily be misled by the omission of detailed information about massage licensing requirements when course materials include massage techniques. Such students may imagine that they could use massage to treat their clients with essential oils, but this practice is illegal in those states that regulate physical contact between clients and therapists. Thus, aromatherapy schools should not include massage techniques without extensive warnings about those states that require a license to touch.

Some schools include introductory massage techniques in their curriculum without sufficiently warning students that a license is required to touch a client in most states and cities in the US. Texas requires a minimum of 300 educational training hours before granting massage licenses, whereas the majority of states require a minimum of 500 hours. The latter states include Arkansas, Connecticut, Delaware, District of Columbia, Florida, Iowa, Louisiana, Maine, Maryland, Missouri, North Carolina, Oregon, Rhode Island, South Carolina, Tennessee, Virginia, Washington, and West Virginia. States requiring between 600 and 750 hours include Alabama, Hawaii, New Hampshire, New Mexico, North Dakota, and Wisconsin. States requiring 1000 or more hours include Nebraska, New York and Utah.[60] In states that do not require a massage license to touch a client, such as for example the state of California, licensing requirements are handled at the local and city level.

The language and choice of examples, questions, case studies, lecture notes and other materials used by aromatherapy schools should reflect the audience for which they are intended, so as to avoid misdirecting students. For example, some curricula include questions like "What essential oil would you choose to treat patients with high blood pressure?" This type of question might misguide students into believing they can "treat" such serious conditions. If the course is designed to teach practicing nurses and physicians how to incorporate essential oils into their professional practices, such a question might be appropriate. However, it is completely unsuitable for an audience with no medical background and no professional basis to treat these conditions. If the intent of the question is simply to caution non-medical students that essential oils exhibit hypertensive or hypotensive actions, the question must be rephrased.

To raise the standards of education, we must also consider the background of aromatherapy instructors. Ideally, there would be national guidelines defining the training needed for aromatherapy teachers. However, until such rigorous standards are formulated, schools and educators should be required to reveal the educational background and professional training of their teachers. Some schools make inflated claims for marketing purposes, so efforts should be made to ensure that their claims are backed by fact. NAHA already has similar requirements for their membership directory; in order to be listed as aromatherapists, members must submit copies of their certificates to the association. Teacher qualification seems a task better suited to the ARC than for NAHA; the ARC could become an aromatherapy teacher registration board also.

A further consideration for raising the educational standards of aromatherapy in the United States relates to continuing education, to ensure that practitioners keep up to date with the latest aromatherapy developments. As NAHA's Council of Schools and Educators and the ARC's Steering Committee raise entry level educational standards, these organizations also will have to develop guidelines for advanced and continuing education.

Training in communication skills is missing in both traditional medical schools and holistic aromatherapy schools, but the principles of holism particularly dictate that practitioners cultivate listening skills to discern the conditions leading to their clients' discomforts or imbalances. If students already have backgrounds as holistic healers, they may have already mastered this art of listening and discerning; most medical practitioners aspiring to incorporate aromatherapy into their repertoire of treatment require greater training in the unquantifiable areas of holistic aromatherapy. As recognized by the present exemption given to students with medical backgrounds, non-medical aromatherapy students require more education in scientific knowledge. Yet medical practitioners searching to incorporate holistic aromatherapy into their practices may require a greater emphasis on the un-measurable skills of synergies, blending, and the role of intuition in emotional and psycho-spiritual balance. The practice of holistic aromatherapy requires instruction in holistic principles and techniques in its core curriculum.

Finally, there is the consideration of practical experience beyond the currently required case studies. Skilled holistic aromatherapists blend oils to suit the particular needs of each patient. In addition to treating patients' physical or emotional complaints, the blended oils must work well together aesthetically. The knowledge, awareness, and listening skills to create these unique individual synergies involve sensitivity and intuition; although basic techniques can be learned through a course of study, mastery of these skills only comes with practice. Ideally, as existing educational standards improve, courses preparing students to become professional aromatherapists will require practical qualifying experience.

The Economics of Aromatherapy

One has only to focus on the stress-reducing effects of aromatherapy to recognize the potential economic benefits. Numerous studies have shown that essential oils reduce stress and anxiety levels, either used alone in inhalations or combined with a massage.[61] Researchers at the American Institute of Stress estimate that 75-90 percent of all visits to health-care providers result from stress-related disorders, and recommend aromatherapy as a beneficial practice for the reduction of stress.[62]

The idea that emotions affect health by acting on neuroendocrine and immune systems has attracted increasing support during the last couple of decades. Recent research in psychoneuro-immunology (PNI) shows that reduction of stress levels reduces disease. Proposing a biomolecular basis for emotions, neuroscientist Candace Pert formulated the concept of body-mind, that admits no separation between body and mind. Her work suggests that "no state of mind exists that is not reflected by a state of the immune system."[63]

Consider the cost savings possible by aromatherapeutic stress relief in prevention of tuberculosis. In 1998, at a meeting of the Psychoneuro-immunology (PNI) Research Society in Bristol, UK, it was reported that tuberculosis is reactivated by stress.[64] According to *London Health*, tuberculosis kills more people around the world than either AIDS or malaria. They estimate a cost of fifty thousand pounds a year to take care of each person suffering from this disease.[65] The state of Georgia in the United States reports an annual average cost of $18,925 per patient[66] while the state of Illinois reports a cost of $68,578 per completed treated case.[67]

Many other studies have also documented the connections between stress and disease. In 1991, Cohen, Tyrell, and Smith studied the relationship between psychological stress and the frequency of documented clinical colds among subjects exposed to respiratory viruses. They found a direct connection between those who caught colds and the levels of stress experienced by these subjects. (Psychological stressors are events that make subjects feel as if their lives were unpredictable, uncontrollable, or overwhelming.)[68] This study also proved that psychological stressors impact the immune system.

Millions of Americans and billions of others around the world succumb to common colds or to influenza viruses with every change in season. They incur medical bills, spending billions of dollars on medication, miss work or school, and their productivity is reduced. Although significant anecdotal evidence points to the anti-viral properties of certain essential oils, there is inadequate substantiated research to base a program of cold prevention on essential oils alone.[69] However, other factors contribute to the common cold or flu besides mere exposure to pathogens. A weakened immune system is an invitation to viruses to invade the body and produce disease. Holistic aromatherapy can assist not only by producing a positive psycho-immune response by stress reduction, but also by strengthening the immune system directly.[70] In combination with a healthy diet, sufficient rest and exercise, certain essential oils can assist in the prevention of the common cold and flu, offering vast cost savings to individuals and society alike.

Other common conditions with similar economic costs are chronic pain, including pre-menstrual and menstrual discomfort. These conditions have similar economic impact on society by impairing productivity and generating medical expenditures, but holistic aromatherapy can assist in cost-effective treatment of these conditions. Chronic pain affects some 80 million Americans, at a cost of approximately $70 billion per year. Jane Buckle reports that the relaxation effects of aromatherapy alone play a role in the management of chronic pain. She further argues that ample evidence supports the use of essential oils as a complementary therapy in the care of patients with chronic pain.[71] Pre-menstrual discomfort such as mood swings, abdominal cramps, and anxiety can also be ameliorated with the use of essential oils.[72] Holistic aromatherapy can ameliorate these symptoms, resulting in tremendous benefits in terms of cost savings and labor productivity.

However, there is more to the economics of aromatherapy than potential cost savings alone. Ecological concerns such as the deforestation being experienced by countries like Madagascar due to the demand for aromatic plants and their products must be considered.[73] Demand for essential oils offers economic opportunities to farmers, especially in developing countries. But mushrooming demands for essential oils pose the danger that wild herbs and aromatic plants may be hunted into extinction, if conservation measures are not observed. Given the political and socioeconomic structures of these countries, these opportunities may benefit only a few people, while exacerbating the abuse of others. Expanding popularity and the possibility for quick returns invite unethical behavior and adulteration of oils for profit. Fair-trade pricing, sustainable farming methods, and potentially healthier societies from the use of less expensive grassroots aromatherapy treatments may outweigh these negative factors. However, more information is necessary to enable more precise cost-benefit analyses, and we who enjoy the advantages of essential oil therapies in the advanced countries should remain conscious of our indebtedness to those third-world countries which often provide the raw materials for aromatherapy.

Conclusions

The future of holistic aromatherapy rests on gaining recognition and acceptance by gathering more knowledge about essential oils and their effects through scientific research with better methodology. Anecdotal evidence needs to be compiled, documented, and, wherever possible, tested. Historical information that elucidates the psycho-spiritual aspects of aromatherapy must be revisited and taught. At the same time, we must bring consumers into the equation by listening to their needs and educating them on the benefits and risks associated with the use of essential oils. Educational standards must continue to improve; organizations like NAHA and ARC must work to assure product labeling and uniformity, and quality public education. In raising the standards of holistic aromatherapy practice, there is a need to unify today's fragmented techniques, to learn from nature's organic complexity and wisdom. Finally, we must be sensitive to ecological issues, and protect nature itself, without which we would not enjoy the healing gifts of aromatherapy in the first place.

Acknowledgments

Special thanks to Gabriel Mojay and Tony Burfield for their valuable input, suggestions, and editorial comments. Much gratitude goes to NAHA Presidents Cheryl Hoard and Jade Shutes, and members of her team, Julia Meadows and Mary Martin, who provided information about NAHA for this chapter. Their dedication and love for aromatherapy have brought NAHA to its current level of professionalism.

Notes

1. Mojay G, *Aromatherapy for Healing the Spirit.* London: Gaia Books Limited, 1996, p. 9.

2. Tisserand, R.B., ed. and trans. *Gattefossé's Aromatherapy.* London: C. W. Daniel, 1937 & 1995.

3. Valnet, J., M.D. *The Practice of Aromatherapy.* London: Healing Arts, 1990.

4. Incomplete essential oils are those from which certain constituents have been removed.

5. Maury, M. *Marguerite Maury's Guide to Aromatherapy, The Secret of Life and Youth: A Modern Alchemy.* London: C. W. Daniel, 1961.

6. Tisserand, R.B., ed. and trans. *Gattefossé's Aromatherapy.* London: C. W. Daniel, 1937 & 1995.

7. McMahon C., "Regardless of one's place on the (spiritual) evolutionary ladder, the lotus (absolute) always leads to higher evolution." "In Search of the White Lotus – Journey to India"; *Aromatic Thymes*, Fall 1998, 6(3): 28.

8. De Groot A. C., and Weyland J. W. "Contact allergy to tea tree oil" *Contact Dermatitis. 1993,* 28: 309. cf. Schaller M., Korting H.C., "Allergic airborne contact dermatitis from essential oils used in aromatherapy." *Clinical and Experimental Dermatology,* 1995, 20(2): 143–145, and Selvaag E., Erikson, B., and Thune, O. "Contact allergy due to tea tree and cross-sensitization to colophony" *Contact Dermatitis*; 1994, 31: 124–125.

9. Sheppard-Hanger S., Lisin G., Watt M., Moyler D. *The Aromatherapy Practitioner Reference Manual,* The Atlantic Institute of Aromatherapy, 1995, p. 67.

10. Ibid., p. 65.

11. Valnet's *Practice of Aromatherapy* includes rosemary, fennel, hyssop, lavender stoechas, wormwood, and sage as epilepsy-inducing oils.

12. Sheppard-Hanger, S., et al., p. 65.

13. Ibid.

14. Battaglia, S. *The Complete Guide to Aromatherapy*, Sydney, Australia: The Perfect Potion, p. 135.

15. Sheppard-Hanger, S., et al., p. 56.

16. Ibid., p. 58

17. Ibid., p. 60.

18. Ibid., pp. 54-55.

19. NAHA Committees Reports, 1998–1999.

20. Schnaubelt K., *Medical Aromatherapy*, Frog, 1999, p. 225.

21. Von Frohlic, E., (1968) "A review of clinical, pharmacological and bacteriological research into Oleum spicae." *Weiner Medizinische Wochenschrift*, 1968, 15, 345–350. cf., Boyd E. M., and Sheppard E. P. "Nutmeg oil and camphene as inhaled expectorants," *Archives of Otolaryngology*, 1970, 92(4): 372–378.

22. Rees, W. D., Evans, B. K., and Rhodes, J. "Treating irritable bowel syndrome with peppermint oil" *British Medical Journal*, 1979, (6194): 835–836. cf., Carle, R., and Gomma, K., "The medicinal use of Matricariae flos" *British Journal of Phytotherapy*, 1992, 2(4): 147–153, and Al-Zuhair, H., Wl-Sayeh, B., Ameen, H. A., and Al-Shoora H. "Pharmacological studies of cardamom oil in animals" *Pharmacological Research*, 1996, 34(1/2): 79–82.

23. Boyd, E. M., and Sheppard, E. P. "The effect of steam inhalation of volatile oils on the output and composition of respiratory tract fluid" *Journal of Pharmacology and Experimental Therapeutics*, 1968, 163(1), 250–256.

24. Guba, R., "Wound Healing—a pilot study using an essential oil based cream to heal dermal wounds and ulcers," *International Journal of Aromatherapy*, 1999, 9(2): 67–74. cf., Glowania, H. J., Raulin, C., and Swododa, M., "Effect of chamomile on wound healing—a clinical double-blind study," *Zeitschrift fur Hautkrankheiten*, 1987, 62(17): 1262, 1267–71.

25. Tisserand R. A*romatherapy to Heal and Tend the Body*, London:Lotus Press, 1988, p. 84.

26. Steam inhalations can be done in the bath, at a sink, or from any container of hot water.

27. There are many different types of micro diffusers. Some use pumps

with glass nebulizers while others disperse the oils from a container such as a bottle. Common aroma lamps use either a candle or a light bulb to heat essential oils that have been added to water. As this solution gets hot, essential oils and water evaporate into the air and thus can be inhaled. Aroma lamps are used for aromatic purposes only as the excessive heat is said to change the molecular structure of essential oils and to render their therapeutic actions ineffective.

28. Damian, P. and K. *Aromatherapy: Scent and Psyche, Using Essential Oils for Physical and Emotional Well-being.* Vermont: Healing Arts Press, 1995.

29. Ludvison, H. W., et al. "Effects of ambient odors of lavender and cloves on cognition, memory, affect and mood," *Chemical Senses,* 1989, 14(4): 525–536.

30. Buchbauer, G., Jirovetz, L., Jager,W., Dietrich, H., and Plank C. "Aromatherapy: evidence for sedative effects of the essential oil of Lavender after inhalation" *Zeitschrift fur Naturforschung Teil C,* 1991, 46(11–12): 1067–1072. cf., Birchall, A. "A Whiff of Happiness" *New Scientist,* 1990, 127(1731): 45–47.

31. Yamaguchi, H. "Effect of odor in heart rate," *The Psychophysiological Effect of Odor,* ed. M. Kouryo., 1990, Tokyo, pp. 168–9.

32. Sugano, H. "Psychophysiological studies of fragrances." In *Fragrance: The Psychology and Biology of Perfume,* Van Toller, S., and Dodd, G. H., eds., 1992, New York: Elsevier Applied Science, pp. 143–161.

33. Birchall, A. "A whiff of happiness," *New Scientist,* 1990, 127(1731): 45–47.

34. Sugano, H., and Sato, N. "Psychophysiological studies of fragrance" *Chemical Senses*,, 1991, 16: 183–184.

35. Lorenzetti, B.B., Souza, G. E., Sarti, S. J., Santos, Filho D., and Ferreira S.H. "Myrcene mimics the peripheral analgesic activity of lemongrass tea" *Journal of Ethnopharmacol,* 1991, 34(1): 43–48. cf., Seth, G., Kokate, C. K., and Varma, K.C. "Effects of Essential Oil of Cymbopogon citratus stapf. on the Central Nervous System," *Indian Journal if Experimental Biology,* 1976, 14(3): 370–371, and Gobel, H., Schmidt, G., and Soyka, D. "Effect of peppermint and eucalyptus oil preparations on neurophysiological and experimental algesimetric headache parameters," *Cephalalgia,* 1994, 14: 228–234.

36. Yousef, R.T. and Tawail, G. C. "Antimicrobial activity of volatile oils;" *Pharmazie,* 1980, 35(11): 698–701. cf. Hinou, J. B., Harvala, C. E., Hinou, E. B., "Antimicrobial activity screening of 32 common constituents of essential oils" *Pharmazie,* 1989, 44(4): 302–303. cf., Dubey, N. K., Kishore, N., and Singh, S. K., "Antifungal properties if the volatile fraction of Melaleuca leucadendron" *Tropical Agriculture,* 1983, 60 (3): 227; Inouye, S. "Antisporulating and respiration-in-

hibitory effects of essential oils on filamentous fungi," *Mycoses,* 1998, 41(9–10): 403–10; and Tadde, I., Giachetti, D., Taddei, F., Mantovani, P., "Spasmolytic activity of Peppermint, Sage and Rosemary essences and their major constituents." *Fitoterapia,* 1988, 59(6): 463–468.

37. Sheppard-Hanger, S. "Percutaneous Confusion or the Evidence on Cutaneous Absorption of Essential Oils," *The World of Aromatherapy,* Frog, 1996, p. 295.

38. Wilkinson, S. "Aromatherapy and massage in palliative care" *International Journal of Palliative Nursing,* 1995, 1(1): 21–30.

39. Stevenson, C. "The psychophysiological effects of aromatherapy massage following cardiac surgery." *Complementary Therapies in Medicine,* 1994, 2: 27–35.

40. "Mean and minty," *New Scientist,* Nov. 1999; previously reported in *Bioresource Technology,* 71: 267.

41. Dube, S., Upadhyay, P. D., and Tripathi, S. C. "Antifungal, physiochemical, and insect–repelling activity of the essential oil of Ocimum basilicum" *Canadian Journal of Botany,* 1989, 67(7): 2085–2087.

42. Ansari, M. A., and Razdan, R.K. "Relative Efficacy of Various Oils in Repelling Mosquitoes" *Indian Journal of Malariology,* 1995, 32(3): 104–111.

43. Watanabe, K., Shono, Y., Kakimizu,A., Okada, A., Matsuo, N., Satoh, A., and Nishimura, H. "New Mosquito Repellent from *Eucalyptus camaldulensis*" *Journal of Agriculture and Food Chemistry,* 1993, 41(11): 2164–2166.

44. Chamberland M., *Annales de l' Institut Pasteur,* 1887, 1:153.

45. Maruzella, J. C., Sicurella, N. A. "Antibacterial activity of essential oils vapors," *Journal of American Pharmaceutical Association,* 1960, 49(11): 693–5.

46. Battaglia, S. "The Role of Research and Science in Aromatherapy," *Aromatherapy Today,* 1999, 11(9): 22–24.

47. Burfield T. "Safety issues in Aromatherapy: the importance of Scientific Data and how it can be properly accessed and assessed." *Proceedings of NAHA World of Aromatherapy II, 1998,* pp. 63–93.

48. Ibid., pp. 63–93.

49. Schnaubelt, K. *Advanced Aromatherapy,* Vermont: Healing Arts Press, 1998, p.17.

50. National Association of Holistic Aromatherapy, *Practitioners and Source Directory, 1999.*

51. Baker, Sylvia. "The Profession, Standards and Safety of Oils," *Positive Health (positivehealth.com)*.

52. Ibid.

53. Jones, L. "Establishing Standards for Essential Oils and Analytical Standards." *Proceedings of NAHA World of Aromatherapy II*, 1998, p. 291.

54. Bascuñana, E. S., *La Nueva Aromaterapia*, Spain: Ediciones Obelisco, p.23.

55. Personal discussion with the Chairperson of the TAP committee, Ms. Julia Meadows, March 29, 2000.

56. www.naha.org, Committee Report.

57. Directory of Schools and Educators, NAHA, Jan. 2000.

58. Personal communication with Jade Shutes, President of NAHA and chairperson of Educational Committee.

59. Press Release provided by ARC Chairperson, Dorene Petersen, and personal conversations with NAHA President, Jade Shutes.

60. Associated Bodywork and Massage Professionals web page, http://www.abmp.com/career.htm #National & Regional Accrediting Agencies.

61. Buckle, J., "Does it matter which lavender essential oil is used?" *Nursing Times*, 1993, 89(20): 32-35. cf. Burns, E., Blamey, C., "Soothing scents in childbirth." *International Journal of Aromatherapy*, 1994, 6: 24-8; Corner, J., Cawley, N., Hilderbrand, S., "An evaluation of the use of essential oils on the wellbeing of cancer patients." *International Journal of Palliative Nursing*, 1995, 1 (2): 67-73; Dunn, C., Sleep, J., Collett, D., "Sensing an improvement—an experimental study to evaluate the use of aromatherapy, massage and periods of rest in and intensive care unit." *Journal of Advanced Nursing*, 1995, 21 (1): 34-40; Miyake, Y., Nakagawa, M., Asakura, Y., "Effects of odors on humans (I). Effects on sleep latency." *Chemical Senses*, 1991, 16: 183; Nagai, H., Nakagawa, M., Nakamura, M., Fujii, W., Inui, T., Asakura, Y., "Effects of odors on humans (II). Reducing effects of mental stress and fatigue." *Chemical Senses*, 1991, 16: 198; Stevenson, C., "The psychophysiological effects of aromatherapy massage following cardiac surgery." *Complementary Therapies in Medicine*, 1994, 2: 27-35; Tasev, T., Toleva, P., Ballabanova, V., "The neuro-psychic effect of Bulgarian rose, lavender and geranium." *Folia Medica*, 1969, 11: 307-17; and Waldman, C. S., Tseng, P., Meulman, P., Whittet, H. B. "Aromatherapy in the intensive care unit." *Care of Critically Ill*, 1993, 9 (4): 170-174.

62. The American Institute of Stress: http://www.stress.org.

63. Pert, C., *Why You Feel the Way You Feel: Molecules of Emotion*. New York:

Scribner, 1997, p. 162.

64. "Evidence for mind-body connection increases." *The Lancet*, April 18, 1998, (351): 9110.

65. http://www.londonhealth.co.uk/tbthreat.asp News 24/3/99

66. DHR Office of Communications – "Tuberculosis in Georgia." May, 1999.

67. Wurts, R., White, W. D., "The cost of tuberculosis: utilization and estimated charges for the diagnosis and treatment of tuberculosis in a public health system." *International Journal of Tuberculosis and Lung Disease*, 1999, 3(5): 382-7.

68. Cohen, S., Tyrell, D. A. J., & Smith, A. P., "Psychological stress and susceptibility to the common cold."*New England Journal of Medicine*, 1991, 325: 606-612.

69. Lembke, A., Deininger, R., "Wirking von Terpenen auf mikroskopische Pilze, Bakterien und Viren," *Phytotherapis, Grundlagen-Klinik-Praxis*, Stuttgart, 1987. cf. Hayashi, K., Kamiya, M., Hayashi, T., "Virucidal Effects of the Steam Distillate from *Houttuynia cordata* and its Components on HSV-1, Influenza Virus and HIV." *Planta Medica*, 1995, 61 (3): 237-241; Cohen, R. A., Kucera, L. S., Herrmann, E. C. Jr., "Antiviral activity of Melissa officinalis," *Proceedings of the Society for Experimental Biology and Medicine*, 1964, 117: 431-4.

70. Pénoël, D. & R., *Natural Home Health Care Using Essential Oils*. Utah: Essential Science Publishing, 1998, pp. 55-60. cf. Mailhebiau, P., *Portraits in Oils – The Personality of Aromatherapy and Their Link with Human Temperaments*, London: C. W. Daniel, 1995, pp. 124-129; Balz, R., *The Healing Power of Essential Oils*. Lotus Light–Shangri-La, 1996, pp. 55-60; Schnaubelt, K., *Medical Aromatherapy*. Frog, 1999, pp. 226-255.

71. Buckle, J., "Use of aromatherapy as a complementary treatment for chronic pain." *Alternative Therapies, Health and Medicine*, September 1999, 5 (5): 42-51.

72. Schnaubelt, K., *Medical Aromatherapy*, Frog, 1999, pp. 254-255.

73. Black, J., "Lecture notes." *Essential oil trader*. Aroma Trading, Ltd., 1998.

Not Just an Apple a Day

Researching and Regulating Medicinal Herbs and Plants

8.

The Potential of Modern Phytotherapy as a Whole-System Science

Dan Kenner, L. Ac.

Introduction

For what kinds of patients does phytotherapy work most reliably?

Botanical medicine, or phytotherapy, is the most widespread form of medical treatment in the world. The World Health Organization (WHO) estimates that 80 percent of the world's population relies principally on traditional medicines, in which phytotherapy plays a central role.[1] Traditional Chinese Medicine (TCM), with its numerous variants, is the most pervasive form of medical therapy in East Asia. Even in Japan, 70 percent of physicians prescribe botanical formulas from *Kampo*, or Chinese medical tradition.[2] In the industrialized West, the use of herbs and botanical extracts plays an increasing role in health care. In France alone, somewhere between 3000 and 4000 physicians use phytotherapy for primary care. Great Britain licenses "Medical Herbalists." German medical schools teach phytotherapy. In the U.S., the sale of herbs is undergoing significant growth. Sales of herbal medicines increased 59 percent in 1997 and are growing 20 percent a year, with the largest growth of sales in retail pharmacies.[3] According to Landmark Health Care of Sacramento, California, herbal therapy has the highest utilization rate of all alternative health care in the U.S., at 17 percent. Among the people surveyed, 70 percent say that they are most likely to use herbal therapy.

Because of this renaissance of interest in phytotherapy in the industrialized West, there has been an increase in clinical research to determine which herbs "work" for which diseases. The issue of how to evaluate herbal efficacy raises larger issues of how patients are initially evaluated and how herbs are selected for prescription.

Traditional herbal methods individualize herbal prescriptions according to a "functional" nosology, organizing signs and symptoms in terms of physiological activities. For example, Chinese medicine uses the term "Spleen *qi* (energy)" to describe physiological activities like peristalsis, digestive absorption, and the circulation of lymph. Conventional allopathic ontological-localized nosology of disease names is not necessarily relevant to this "functional" diagnosis. The ontological-localized nosology classifies a disorder as a lesion or anomaly within a given anatomical system. A typical example is a gastric ulcer, consisting of a lesion (ulceration) in a locus (stomach). But Chinese practitioners would not be guided by this lesion/location diagnosis in their phytotherapy evaluation. The relevant Chinese functional nosological entities might be "Spleen dampness," "Spleen *qi* vacuity," or "Liver *qi* congestion."[4]

But each of these Chinese nosologies, like all functional classifications, is a disorder of the patient's entire physiology. "Spleen dampness" might indicate mucous membrane hypersecretion. A "Spleen vacuity," in Western terms, could mean an enzyme deficiency or immune system disorder. "Liver *qi* congestion" might indicate biliary dyskinesia or a psychogenic disorder. But each of these Chinese diagnostic categories can have a variety of manifestations. For example, spleen dampness can manifest as gastrointestinal disorders, arthritic disorders, bronchitis, or even epilepsy. From the Chinese viewpoint, what is at issue is not merely a lesion in the location where it happens to appear, but the redressing of a dangerous imbalance that might lead to other symptoms if balance is not reestablished. Diagnosis of these functional conditions in all cases requires a thorough history and physical examination. New research strategies in Japan and China have endeavored to compensate for this dissonance between holistic and reductionistic paradigms.

Prospective Research

> "Nobody likes to ask if a model is really correct, since if they did, most work would have come to a halt."
> —Francis Crick, *What Mad Pursuit*, 1988

The double-blind placebo-controlled study is the gold standard for determining efficacy in the evaluation of drugs. In fact, double-blind paradigms are fraught with uncertainty.[5] There are also questions about the scientific definition of a placebo.[6] And although double-blind placebo-controlled studies supposedly determine pharmaceutical drugs to be safe and effective, the frequency at which they have been subjected to review (nearly 50 percent) and even taken off the market casts doubt on the scientific infallibility of this standard. It is likely, however, that the double-blind placebo-controlled study will maintain its status for the foreseeable future. Newer methods of evaluation such as outcome studies are acceptable to the academically oriented, but are less acceptable to more conservative government regulatory bodies.

Botanical medicines are not only marketed but also included in the National Health Insurance systems in Japan and France. Yet it has seemed economically unwise for herbal manufacturers to do controlled clinical trials of their products. Controlled studies that could yield negative results are avoided as unnecessary risks, since the game is rigged to their disadvantage. The conventional profession complains, "Why don't they want to test their medications? What have they got to hide?" But no single herb is effective for treating all patients, of different genetic types, different etiologies, and different physiological parameters. Because of the paucity of clinical trials, some National Health Insurance coverage has been reduced, but this has not stopped the Japanese or the French from being among the highest consumers of herbal products in the world.

China has integrated modern research methodology with holistic prescription systems. Chinese diagnostic criteria are identical to the WHO criteria for hypertension, a Western diagnostic entity.

Then Chinese practice subdivides these patients into subcategories like: "Exuberance of liver fire," "Vacuity of yin with an exuberance of yang," "Vacuity of yin and yang," or "Accumulation of phlegm-dampness." Chinese hepatitis studies evaluate all patients with standard blood tests for liver enzymes and antibodies. Then clinical evaluation subdivides the population into groups of "Spleen vacuity with invasion of toxicity," "Damp-heat of liver and spleen," "Vacuity of yin with heat in the blood," and "Blood stagnation and obstruction in the liver channel." Cerebral vascular accident is subdivided into no less than nine different diagnostic categories.[7] Each category of diagnosis indicates a different type of herbal prescription. As results are obtained, they are collated and evaluated collectively according to "Western" diagnoses.

In Japan, similar attempts to individualize treatment in research design were met with suspicion. Despite good initial media coverage, the medical community disparaged individualized treatment with different herbal formulas according to the patient's symptom-sign complex as lacking controls and rigorous research design. Despite such criticism, the Japanese results were good enough to get the attention of researchers who did further studies using more reductionistic research designs.

Unfortunately there have been some negative effects from using the same herb formula for *all* patients with hepatitis C or liver cirrhosis. For example, the herb bupleurum (*Bupleurum falcatum*) contains saikosaponins *a*, *b*, *c* and *d*. Saikosaponin *b* has been shown especially effective for treating intractable chronic hepatitis.[9] Minor Bupleurum Combination contains ginseng (*Panax ginseng*), which contains saponins that protect liver cells from carbon tetrachloride-induced hepatotoxicity and accelerate regeneration of liver cells.[11] Minor Bupleurum Combination also contains licorice (*Glycyrrhiza glabra*) which increases interferon production. Glycyrrhizin, an active compound of licorice, has been used intravenously for chronic hepatitis B and has caused complete recoveries on occasion.[10] Another ingredient of Minor

Bupleurum Combination is Scute, also called Chinese skullcap (*Scutellaria baicalensis*), which has been shown to stimulate the production of interleukins (IL-5, IL-6 and IL-10) in hepatitis C patients.[12] So based on laboratory science criteria, Minor Bupleurum Combination seemed a good candidate for a "one-size-fits-all" hepatitis treatment.[8]

However, four patients taking Minor Bupleurum Combination for chronic hepatitis C developed interstitial pneumonitis, possibly caused by interferon or the combination of interferon with the formula. Interstitial pneumonitis is also induced by granulocyte colony-stimulating factors (G-CSF). It was subsequently found that Minor Bupleurum Combination stimulated G-CSF production in peripheral blood mononuclear cells.[13]

Numerous variations of bupleurum-based formulas treat a variety of symptom-sign complexes and types of patients. When immune system mechanisms go into action in the presence of hepatitis B virus, some people recover and others die, not only because of severity of the virus, but because of individual differences in disposing of it. The traditional-style herbalist would ask whether these negative results were caused by a failure to individualize treatment, that damaged the yin in susceptible patients, or by an immune system reaction to mobilizing too many necrotic liver cells at once.

Applying conventional research methodologies to phytotherapy research has created numerous other difficulties. Combinations display different properties than their component herbs, and single herbs behave differently from "active principles."[14] Formulas' synergies depend not only on their combination of herbs but also on their method of preparation. Researchers found that saikosaponins *a* & *d* were not available in Minor Bupleurum Combination, but saikosaponin *b* was abundant.[15] In other bupleurum combinations used to stabilize psychic and nervous system functions, saikosaponins *a* & *d* were available, but not *b*.[15] The synergy of components in the formulas causing different chemical reactions was the explanation for the discrepancies. Researchers found that when they decocted licorice root with coptis root (*Coptidis chinensis*), new compounds were formed that were not present in either herb.

Such synergies of herbal formulas challenge paradigms based on active principles. Most formal attempts to validate herbal medications focus on which chemical components are active for certain symptoms or diseases. Researchers found that serum levels of the active principle of *Ma Huang* (*Ephedra sinensis*), ephedrine, were higher in patients that had been given *Ma Huang* and Apricot Seed Combination than in patients that were given pure ephedrine.[16] Serum ephedrine levels were obtained when *Ma Huang* was decocted in the traditional formula *Ma Huang* and Gypsum Decoction with no new compounds formed from the decoction process.[17] Licorice was found to potentiate the activity of the ephedra even though it decreased the plasma level of ephedrine.

So there is a need for methods of testing appropriate to botanical medication. Ignoring the details of personal history and physical examination will neither validate the traditional uses of herbs nor develop their therapeutic potential. When traditional formulas were reintegrated into the health care system in Japan in the early 1970s, the Japanese Medical Association took the position that conventional diagnostic methods were not sensitive enough to make prescriptions of traditional formulas. Prescription of herbal formulas depended on subjective evaluation of the symptoms and signs traditionally associated with the formulas. The use of traditional formulas was adopted without validation studies because it was believed that modern methods of laboratory evaluation could coexist with the traditional clinical observations.[18] Yet the rewards of developmental research in phytotherapy may be rich.

Several botanical medications show promise in cancer treatment. Previous claims stated that Chinese herbal medicine only prolonged the lives of patients and protected their immune systems. Clinical trials indicated that their cancers were effectively treated with few side effects. The Chinese herbal combination known as PC-SPES proved effective in the treatment of prostate cancer.[20] An intravenous herb drip and oral preparation of the herb *Semen coicis* has been used to induce remission of different types of cancer, especially digestive tract cancers.[21] In Europe as well, intravenous *Chelidonium majus*,[22] *Helleborus niger*,[23] and *Dionaea muscipula*[24] have demonstrated dramatic effects not only in strengthening the function of the immune system, but also in tumor reduction. Doctors in France using a whole-system model are able to individualize diagnosis and use botanical medications to regulate nervous system and endocrine function to a sophisticated degree, treating even disorders like diabetes and hypothyroidism without the use of hormones. They are able to treat even severe infections without antibiotics utilizing the powerful disinfectant properties of essential oils.[19]

Herbal extracts are used in Chinese hospitals for treating cardiovascular disease, autoimmune diseases, bacterial infections, kidney diseases and burns.[25] These breakthroughs in herbal treatment are being made in countries conducting developmental research in treating chronic disease problems with non-toxic therapies.

Standards

In the U.S. today, much of the controversy over herbal products in the marketplace is about standards of quality. The 1994 Dietary Supplement Health and Education Act (DSHEA) classification of herbs, vitamins, minerals, etc. as nutritional or dietary supplements has been criticized for allowing these supplements to be marketed without testing for safety, efficacy, or quality. In fact, the safety definition for dietary supplements is actually stricter for supplements than it is for foods or drugs. Dietary supplements, including herbs, are considered unsafe if they "present a significant or unreasonable risk of illness or injury." By contrast, drugs are permitted to present "significant" risks, as long as risks are outweighed by benefits. By law, statements made about efficacy must be supported by scientific evidence.[26] The U.S. Food and Drug

Administration is required to prove a product unsafe before it can be taken off the market. Regulating agencies in Germany, France, the United Kingdom, Canada, and Japan also enforce standards of herbal product quality, as well as safety assessment of herbal product manufacturers.[27][28]

There remain several uncertainties with regard to standards. Potency of substances is also affected by growing conditions, storage, handling, as well as subsequent methods of preparation. Standards of potency are resolved by standardizing the quantity of an "active principle" of an herbal extract. Critics of standardization claim that destroying the integrity of an herb's natural chemical balance by adding other substances, sometimes synthetic, to standardize the product does not enhance quality.[29]

Another controversy arises over which component is *the* active one. Many herbs have numerous substances that could be deemed "active." We have already seen the problems of "active principle" isolation and interaction in the Bupleurum case above. France's solution confers pharmaceutical grade status on botanical extracts containing minimum levels of all constituents designated pharmacologically active.

Accurate plant identification is another important issue in standards of quality. Mistakes can be made when the wrong part of the plant is used, for the same plant may have parts with very different types of activity. Bogus echinacea has appeared on the market. There have also been cases of fraudulent ginseng labeling.[32] Herbs have also been misidentified with dangerous results, as in the case where belladonna poisoning occurred among consumers of an herbal tea in New York City.[30] In another case digitalis poisoning resulted from ingesting a mislabeled extract of plantain.[31]

Contamination of herbal raw materials can pose a problem. Crude plant substances in warehouses can be subjected to spraying with pesticides. Different countries have different standards regarding agricultural pest control. Pesticides banned in the U.S. are still widely used in other countries. Heavy metal residues in

The Potential of Modern Phytotherapy as a Whole-System Science

Chinese herbal patent medicines have been detected in the U.S., perhaps as a result of pesticide contamination.[33] But it should be noted that many Chinese companies conform to international standards of quality and purity in their manufacturing practices.

France uses high performance liquid chromatography (HPLC) for analysis of components as well as in the detection of contaminants in products designated pharmaceutical grade. The Pharmaceutical Affairs Bureau of Japan's Ministry of Health and Welfare also regulates the quality of botanical formulas, monitoring specific plant constituents so that the herbal ingredients of each formula meet precise standards of quality.[34]

Medical Education

The greatest concern to physicians in the U.S. today is herb-drug interactions; information is limited on the vast variety of herbal products on the market, but it is gradually becoming available. In the U.S., the likelihood of interactions between drugs and herbs is higher than elsewhere because doctors in the U.S. are more likely to prescribe a prescription drug than an herb, compared to Germany or Japan, where many doctors already use alternatives. National health care in Germany and Japan already covers herbal products prescribed by physicians. In the U.S., physicians are beginning to notice that over 60 million Americans use herbs; the number is even higher if other supplements are included. This number is expected to increase, especially in medical use, as insurance companies begin to cover herbal use. It is desirable that all health care providers have some basic knowledge of herbs, but it is also necessary for training to be available for those practitioners who wish to become specialists or experts in phytotherapy. The development of phytotherapy depends on the commitment of interested professionals to go beyond the "specific symptom" approach heavily promoted by manufacturers. This symptomatic approach simplifies the complexity of herbs and extracts into the image of a drug with a single type of application that allegedly benefits all potential users. This one-dimensional approach advocates St. John's Wort (*Hypericum perforata*) for depression, feverfew (*Tanacetum parthenium*) for migraines, or ginger (*Zingiberis officinalis*) for motion sickness.

The complex properties of herbs must be studied and applied within the context of more complex "functional" whole-system models of physiology. These systems are widely used even in official medicine in East Asia, and to a lesser extent in the U.S. and Europe. Whole-system models of clinical practice individualize treatment based on each patient's personal traits, body type, or "terrain," and the "balance" of physiological functions. If an exudative type of patient suffers from bronchitis, then herbs for hypersecretion should be used to dry up the condition. If the patient also suffers fatigue, is elderly, or has low adrenal function, an adrenal stimulant like black currant might be added. If the bronchitis patient has a spasmodic cough with bronchial constriction, a disinfectant substance might be recommended like essential oil of thyme, considered "vagolytic" by French phytotherapy doctors. If the bronchitis patient has a diabetic tendency, oil of eucalyptus, considered to be hypoglycemiant, might be chosen instead.[35] As in French phytotherapy of the terrain, Ayurvedic and Chinese medical systems have long traditions of diagnosis that adjust treatment according to a complex interpretation of symptoms and signs.

It is important to understand these models of phytotherapy as being problem-solving methodologies, or clinical "software," and not merely cultural artifacts or metaphysical ideologies. Although Ayurveda and some systems of Chinese medicine may appear metaphysical, they also contain the elements of patient-centered practice. These systems are taught in China, Japan, India and in some western European nations. In the U.S., many acupuncture specialists study traditional-style Chinese phytotherapy. When successful, a whole-system approach will match the patient's pathophysiology correctly and preclude the possibility of side effects. In

The Potential of Modern Phytotherapy as a Whole-System Science

reality there are no "*side* effects" for any medication. There are only *effects*. The goal of whole-system treatment is to seek the correct combination of herbs to balance out unwanted effects or one-sided effects from individual herbs.

Teaching whole-system models for herbal prescription to practitioners of phytotherapy will gradually produce a population of clinical experts with capabilities beyond the "patent medicine" approach. Instruction in entry-level herbal medicine approaches should be made widely available to practitioners who do not intend to become specialists, but wish to offer the benefits of nontoxic treatment to their patients.

Public Awareness

In the U.S. in recent years, articles have appeared in news media about the dangers of herbs. Alleged hazards are overstated even to the point of "fear propaganda," but the alleged dangers do not appear to represent a public health problem. According to the National Poison Control Center in Atlanta, the rate of occurrence of herbal poisonings is one out of every million. The most frequent causes of herbal poisoning are ingestion of house plants, usually by children, and mushroom poisoning. There have been no poisoning fatalities from commercial products, and fewer than "a half-dozen cases in five years."[36]

By contrast, the fourth leading cause of death in the U.S. is fatalities from prescribed drugs; the number of such deaths exceeds 100,000 a year. Every year, prescription drugs cause 1 million injuries so severe that they require hospitalization; another 2 million drug-related injuries occur *during* hospital care.[37] Dr. Brian Strom, Associate Director of Medicine and Pharmacology at the University of Pennsylvania School of Medicine, estimated that drug side effects result in the hospitalization of 1.6 million people at a cost of more than US $20 billion each year.[50] In a review of one ten-year period by the Government Accounting Office, more than half of newly-approved drugs were recalled due to unexpected side effects—problems that had not yet surfaced during the long and expensive research conducted for the FDA approval process.[38]

These numbers, while horrifying, do not negate the importance of physicians' concerns over herbal safety. Estimated sales of herbal medicine in the U.S. reached $1.2 billion in 1996.[40] According to a survey by Applied Biometrics of North Palm Beach, Florida, 62 percent of American consumers take herbs for disease prevention, 54 percent to increase energy, 40 percent to improve fitness, 31 percent to increase alertness, and 27 percent to reduce stress.[41] Many patients in the U.S. and Europe seek nontoxic "soft" therapy first and use dangerous substances as a backup or last resort. In France, Germany, Japan, and China, physicians have adapted to this strategy. In Japan in the 1960s there was a public uprising, now referred to as the "*Kampo* Boom," when public demand rehabilitated the traditional herbal medicine against the excessive use of pharmaceuticals. Even though this has not solved the problem with the overuse of drugs, it now offers an alternative within the mainstream.[39]

The chief danger of herb use is in additive interactive effects with prescription drugs the patient already is using. Consumers would be well advised to consult with experienced phytotherapy practitioners regarding the long-term use of any botanical substance or combination. Consumers using prescription drugs should obtain medical advice regarding potential problems resulting from herb-drug interactions. Women should exercise special caution if pregnant or lactating. Consumers who are self-medicating using packaged products should shop for those that label the expiration date, lot number, botanical name of the herb, strength of the recommended dose, and the name and address of the manufacturer. No reasonable person would oppose efforts to develop standards, or a grading system for botanical products with respect to their proper identification, potency, safe handling, proper storage, and their influences on pathophysiology. All efforts to do so are salutory, beneficial for the public and for the health care professions.

Cost-Effectiveness

Formal cost-effectiveness studies are rare even in East Asia where the economic impact of herbs in the medical marketplace is greatest. One reason that 10 percent of Americans self-medicate is that herbs are much less expensive than prescription drugs.[42] In Third World nations, drugs are prohibitively expensive for an even larger portion of the population. When an herb can be shown to be as effective as a pharmaceutical drug for a medical disorder, it can be a significant cost reduction factor. In Germany, Bayer Corporation markets St. John's Wort as an antidepressant. In Canada, Nytol maker, the Block Drug Company, sells valerian as a sleep aid, and Johnson & Johnson sells feverfew for migraine treatment. Studies have shown saw palmetto (*Serenoa repens*) berry extract as effective as finisteride for benign prostatic hyperplasia.[43] Herbal medications are potentially effective for withdrawing patients from benzodiazepine drugs, at a significant savings in cost as well as in quality of life.[44] Herbs have also been tested for a variety of other complaints including nausea,[45] hyperglycemia,[47] circulation problems,[48] hypercholesterolemia,[49] and hormone regulation for disorders of climacteric.[46] Thus there is tremendous potential to reduce health care costs by using herbs and herbal extracts.

The use of nontoxic therapies can also be contrasted with the cost-effectiveness of a system based primarily on pharmaceutical drugs. As one counts the miracle drugs that have appeared and disappeared over the history of pharmaceutical companies' producing dangerous products that are later quietly removed from the market, one gets the impression of a serious failure to provide safe, inexpensive care. If we include quality of life issues, the problem is less quantifiable, but no less significant. Drug side effects such as impotence, depression, rashes, dizziness, confusion, and even shortened life span underscore the need to develop an accounting of risks versus benefits that is not just quantitative. These dangers are a significant reason that $11 billion has been spent by 1/3 of Americans on alternative health care.[51]

Education about phytotherapy should include the laboratory-based approach to symptoms and diseases, but should also make use of whole-system clinical models. Efforts to educate the public, the health care professions, and public policy-makers about the integration of botanical medicines into the health care arena should objectively evaluate the costs and benefits of existing pharmaceutical-based medical systems and its acceptability to consumers.

The future development of phytotherapy in world medicine will require new levels of research addressing treatment of cancer, AIDS, cardiovascular diseases, chronic pain, and similar health care problems that most burden public health provider systems. In order to integrate phytotherapy into national health care delivery systems, we face an urgent need to solve problems of quality control standards, efficacy, and third-party payment. Future developments in phytotherapy should include research into cross-cultural comparison of how phytotherapy is integrated into health care systems in different nations.

Notes

1. Saleh, A.A., "La plante medicinale de la tradition a la science." *First International Congress of Clinical Phytotherapy.* Paris: Jacques Grancher, 1997.

2. Ross, C. "New life for old medicine." *Lancet.* 1992, 342: 486-487.

3. *Drug Store News.* "The right stuff: *Drug Store News* picks the categories taking off in '94." 1994, 16: 15.

4. Ellis, Wiseman and Boss. *Fundamentals of Chinese Medicine.* Brookline, MA: Paradigm, 1988.

5. Fisher, S., Greenberg, R., "Second opinion: rethinking the claims of biological psychiatry." *The Limits of Biological treatments for Psychological Distress.* Hillsboro, NJ: Laurence Erlbaum, 1989.

6. Parfitt, Andrew. "Placebo treatments." *Proceedings* of the First Symposium of the Society for Acupuncture Research. Rockville, MD, 1993.

7. *Xinyao Shenpi Banfa* (Provisions for New Drug Approval). Beijing: The Ministry of Public Health, 1985 (In Chinese and English).

8. Abe, H., Arichi, S., et al. *Yakugaku Zasshi* [*Journal of Pharmacology*] 1980, 100(6): 602-610.

9. Li, W., and Lien, E., "A survey of Chinese herbs: *Bupleurum chinense*," *Bulletin of the Oriental Healing Arts Institute.* 1984, 9 (5): 237-245.

10. Sato, H. et al., "Therapeutic basis of glucyrrhizin on chronic hepatitis B."*Antiviral Research* (Toyama Medical and Pharmaceutical University, Japan), May, 1996, 30 (2-3): 171-177.

11. Jeong, T. C., et al., "Protective effects of ginseng saponins against carbon tetrachloride-induced hepatotoxicity in Sprague Dawley rats." (Toxicology Research Center, Korea Research Institute of Chemical Technology, Taejon.) *Planta Med.* April 1997, 63 (2): 136-140.

12. Yamashiki, M. et al., "Effects of Japanese herbal medicine *Sho-saiko-to* (TJ-9) on in vitro interleukin-10 production by peripheral blood mononuclear cells of patients with chronic hepatitis C." *Hepatology* , June 1997, 25 (6): 1390-1397.

13. Ishizaki, T. et al., "Pneumonitis during interferon and/or herbal drug therapy in patients with chronic active hepatitis." *European Respiratory Journal.* Dec. 1996, 9 (12): 2691-2696.

14. Kenner, Dan, & Requena, Yves. *Botanical Medicine: A European Professional Perspective.* Brookline, MA: Paradigm, 1996, p. 18.

15. Kubo, Michinori, *Kampo Iyakugaku.* Tokyo: Kogawa shoten, 1985, pp. 83–86.

16. Kubo Michinori, *Kampo no Rinsho Yakugaku.* Osaka: Kaigai Pub. 1978, p. 37.

17. Hasegawa, M., ed. *Herbal Medicine: Kampo Past and Present.* Tokyo: Tsumura Juntendo, 1985, pp. 52-66.

18. Yakazu, D., "Takemi Kaicho ga Kampo Seizai wo Yakka Kijun ni Tosai no Ketsui wo surumade no Haikei [Background of the decision of inclusion of Kampo drugs in the National Health Insurance by Dr. Takemi, President of the Japanese Medical Association." *Kampo no Rinsho*, 1987, 34 (7): 442-447.

19. Kenner, Dan, & Requena, Yves, as in note 14.

20. Study at Sloan Kettering Memorial cited in *The New Yorker*, October 26, 1998. No completed studies published yet, but studies are under way at the Cancer Research Institute, New York Medical College, Robert Wood Johnson Medical School, and the University of California at San Francisco Cancer Center. Early findings consistently reported PSA levels lowered by 50% and clearance in major metastatic sites.

21. Ye, J. Q., et al., *Jiangsu Zhongyi [Jiangsu Journal of Traditional Chinese Medicine]*. 1962, (1): 29, reports that Zhejiang College of Traditional Chinese Medicine developed "*Kang Lai Te*," patented in China, Russia, the Philippines, and the U.S. for cancer treatment.

22. Nowicky, J. W., et al., "Sensitization for specific lysis in target-effector-systemwith derivatives of *Chelidonium majus L.* alkaloids." Proceedings of the 16th International Congress of Chemotherapy, Ukraine, June 1989, p. 852.

23. Trials underway in Germany.

24. Todorov, D.K. et al., "Antitumor activity of *Dionaea muscipula E.* preparation *Carnivora* new *in vitro* and *in vivo*, on animal and human tumors sensitive and resistant to antitumor drugs," (National Center of Oncology, Sofia, Bulgaria,) *Biotech. & Biotechnol. Eq.*, 1998, 12: 2.

25. Li, C. P. *Chinese Herbal Medicine*, U.S. Dept. HEW, NIH (1974).

26. McCaleb, R. Herbal Research Foundation's response to the *New England Journal of Medicine* editorial of September 17, 1998: www.herbs.org.

27. Tyler, V. E., *Herbs of Choice: The Therapeutic Use of Phytomedicinals*. Binghamton, NY: Pharmaceuticals Products Press, 1994.

28. Newall, C. A., Anderson, L. A., and Phillipson, J. D., *Herbal Medicine: A Guide for Health Care Professionals*. London: Pharmaceutical Press, 1996.

29. Awang, D., "Feverfew trials: The promise of – and problem with – standardized botanical extracts." *Herbalgram*, 1997, (41): 16-17.

30. "Herbal roulette." *Consumer Reports*. November 1995: 698-705.

31. *The Denver Post*. June 13, 1997.

32. Siegel, R. "Kola, ginseng, and mislabeled herbs." *Journal of the American Medical Association*, 1978, 237: 24.

33. Ko, R. "Adulterants in Asian patent medicines," *New England Journal of Medicine*, 1998, 339 (12).

34. Tsutani, K. "Dentoteki Iyakuhin ni tai suru Senshinkoku no Seifu, Seiyakusangyo no yakuwari [Role of the government and the drug industry on traditional drugs in developed countries]." *Rinsho Igaku*, 1988, 4: 855-860

35. Duraffourd, C., Lapraz, J. C., Valnet, J., *ABC de la Phytotherapie dans les maladies infectieuses*. Paris: Jacques Grancher, 1998.

36. Atlanta Poison Control Center.

37. Moore, T., "Prescription for Safety," *Natural Health*, October, 1998, pp. 52-55.

38. *General Accounting Office*, April, 1990.

39. Fukushima, M. "Overdose of drugs in Japan." *Nature*, 1989, 342: 850-851.

40. Tyler, V. E., "What pharmacists should know about herbal remedies." *Journal of the American Pharmacological Association*, 1996, 36: 29-37.

41. *The Business of Herbs*, March/April, 1996, p. 29.

42. Duke, J. "Why people take supplements," *Nature's Herbs*, 1(2).

43. Bach, D., Schmitt, M., and Ebeling, L. "Phytopharmaceutical and synthetic agents in the treatment of benign prostatic hyperplasia (BPH)." *Phytomedicine*, 1997, 3 (4): 309-313.

44. Rasmussen, P. "A role for phytotherapy in the treatment of benzodiazepine and opiate drug withdrawal (part 1)." *The European Journal of Herbal Medicine*, 1997, 3 (1): 11-21.

45. Bone, M. E., et al., "Ginger root: a new antiemetic: the effect of ginger root on postoperative nausea and vomiting after major gynecological surgery." *Anesthesia*, 1990, 45: 669-671.

46. Zava, D. et al., "Estrogen and progestin bioactivity of foods, herbs and spices." *PSEBM*, 1998, 217: 369-378.

47. Yokozawa, T. et al., "Studies on the mechanism of the hypoglycemic activity of ginsenoside-Rb2 in streptozotocin-diabetic rats." *Chem Pharm Bull.* 1985, 14: 255-259.

48. Bauer, U. "Six-month double-blind randomized clinical trial of *Ginkgo biloba* extract versus placebo in two parallel groups in patients suffering from peripheral arterial insufficiency." *Arzneim Forsch Drug Res.* 1984, 34 (1): 716-720.

49. Aue, W. et al., "Hypertension and hyperlipidemia: garlic helps in mild cases." *Brit. J Clin Pract.* 1990, 69: 3-6.

50. Strom, B., "As prescription drugs cure, some side effects harm," *Philadelphia Inquirer*, June 24, 1990.

51. *Natural Pharmacy*, Oct/Nov 1996, 1 (1).

9.
Phytotherapy
Challenges for the 21st Century

Kerry Bone
Fellow, National Institute of Medical Herbalists (UK)
Fellow, National Herbalists Association of Australia

The field of phytotherapy is facing some major challenges as we move into the 21st century. These issues exist now and are likely to significantly shape the future use of plants as therapeutic agents throughout the world. Drawing on my experience as both a phytotherapist and consultant for an herbal manufacturer, I would like to offer my perspective on the following significant challenges:

- The challenge of proof.
- The challenge posed by misinformation.
- The challenge of safety regulation.
- The challenge of quality.
- The challenge of disease prevention.
- The challenge of the patient.
- The challenge of sustainability.

The Challenge of Proof

It is vital that we improve the quality of evidence that herbal medicines work. However, part of this task also lies in demonstrating that existing traditional information constitutes an appropriate level of proof in many circumstances.

Information about the use of an herb comes from the following sources:

- Traditional use.
- Scientific studies—both pharmacological and clinical.
- Folk use.
- Anecdotal accounts.

The concept of traditional knowledge is very poorly understood even among some phytotherapists and herbalists. Conventional medical scientists commonly confuse traditional use information with that of folk use or anecdotal accounts. It is important that herbalists and phytotherapists elevate the concept of traditional use to the high status it deserves. To do so, we must exercise some intellectual rigor in establishing what does and what does not constitute real traditional knowledge. "Real tradition" exists in the context of a traditional medical system that has evolved over thousands of years—or it may be part of a smaller or more primitive system. The important point is that valid traditional use is knowledge refined over many generations, carefully evaluated and re-evaluated by many of the practitioners of the craft. It is not just the anecdotal accounts of a few practitioners. When traditional use is part of a great system and culture, the information therein should be rated highly because it has evolved over many years and been tried on large numbers of people. The great systems of herbal medicine are Ayurveda, Unani, Traditional Chinese Medicine and Western Herbal Medicine. In this context, traditional knowledge represents a cumulative wisdom that overrides aberrations from so-called placebo effects and observer bias. This is not to say that such traditional use data should not also be critically evaluated and reviewed, because it is just as possible for myths to be perpetuated in traditional systems as they are perpetuated in scientific systems.

An important value of traditional use data is that it can be used, where appropriate, to guide scientific exploration. For example, Echinacea contains polysaccharides that *in vitro* experiments have found to stimulate some aspects of immune function. Since ethanol will not extract polysaccharides, this has led some writers to conclude that high ethanolic extracts of Echinacea are inactive. This is despite the fact that most of the traditional use data comes from the Eclectics who used an 80 percent ethanolic extract. This arrogant disregard for traditional data will only lead to misinformation and blind allies.

A good example of how respect for traditional knowledge can guide and enhance scientific research is provided in a recent publication on the traditional Incan medical herb, cat's claw. Professor Klaus Keplinger of Austria has been studying *Uncaria tomentosa* (cat's claw) for many years; his team has been granted several patents concerning the immune activity of some of the cat's claw's constituents. Now his group has published a study that contains the results of their extensive ethnomedical, botanical, pharmacological and toxicological research. There is even a pilot clinical study described in the paper.[1]

The medicinal system of the Asháninka Indians of Peru is first portrayed. Three categories of medical disorders and healers are recognized. A human is viewed to consist of a physical and a spiritual being who communicate with each other by means of a regulating element. The Asháninka expression of "I am healthy" literally means "I carry harmony." The significance of cat's claw in their traditional medicine is emphasized by its exclusive use by priests to influence this regulation, which is regarded as a spiritual matter. The priests are the highest level of healers who adhere to a vegetarian diet and are appointed after years of education by their mentors in complete seclusion in the forests.

Keplinger's group has found that there are two chemotypes of cat's claw. (Chemotypes or chemical races are races within a plant species that are normally indistinguishable but produce different phytochemicals.) One chemotype contains pentacyclic oxindole alkaloids (POA) and the other contains both POA and tetracyclic indole and oxindole alkaloids (TOA). Supernatants of endothelial cell cultures incubated with low levels of POA increase the proliferation of normal resting or weakly activated human B and T lymphocytes. The POA do not directly influence the proliferation, but rather induce endothelial cells to release an unidentified factor which influences the proliferation of lymphocytes. In contrast, TOA act antagonistically on the release of this factor.

Thirteen patients with HIV infection who refused to receive other therapies took an extract of cat's claw root (the chemotype containing only POA) for 2.2 to 5.0 months. Although the total white blood cell count remained unchanged within the group, it was found that low values were raised and high values were lowered. The lymphocyte count increased significantly by an average of around 35 percent. However, no significant changes of T4 to T8 cell ratios were observed.

In their discussion, the authors emphasize that the use of cat's claw must take into account that at least two chemotypes of the plant exist. These are distinguished by the Asháninka priests who exclusively harvest the POA-type plants—but it is a mystery how the priests achieve this selectivity. Keplinger continues:

"The question of chemotype is especially important when antagonistic effects are to be expected from the wrong type, as in the case of *U. tomentosa*. This fact has been widely ignored by today's manufacturers who have never asked a native authority. We analyzed some fifty 'uña de gato' or cat's claw products from the United States, Central America and Peru and found varying mixtures of pentacyclic and tetracyclic (up to 80 percent of total) alkaloids."

This landmark study demonstrates that scientific research which respects traditional insights can not only lead to new pharmacological developments, but can also shed additional light on traditional practices. While the pentacyclic oxindole alkaloids are probably not the only active components in cat's claw, the selection of the POA chemotype by the native authorities strongly suggests that it should be preferred. The use of the correct chemotype will further advance our understanding of this important herb.

Clearly more clinical trials of herbs are needed. At present in the western world, the majority of trials are funded by corporations. It is critical that governments recognize the widespread usage of herbal medicines in their communities and make funds available for clinical research. America's National Institute of Health is already making such funds available. The design of a good clinical trial is very difficult, and there are many texts and articles on this subject. Accordingly, trials on herbs should be very critically assessed. Results from open trials (lacking control groups) or trials which are not double blind should only be regarded as preliminary.

Folk use and anecdotal information should be treated with skepticism by the herbal reader. Folk use is here defined to mean small-scale use, often in an isolated context, and should therefore not be confused with traditional use. For example, the book by Maria Treben is an example of folk use, whereas the British Herbal Pharmacopoeia 1983 documents traditional use. That is not to say that folk use data and anecdotal information are without value, but rather that they should be considered hypothetical rather than proven.

The Challenge Posed by Misinformation

Probably the quickest and easiest way to research medicinal plants is to use some form of *in vitro* test. The literal meaning of the term *in vitro* is "in glass"; it typically refers to laboratory experiments conducted on isolated animal or human cell cultures, microorganisms, enzyme systems, or pharmacological receptors. While *in vitro* research can be very useful—for example it may establish possible antibacterial or antiviral activity—it has a number of limitations. These limitations particularly apply in the field of herbal research, because herbs are usually administered orally, are chemically complex, and consist entirely of natural products often with unknown pharmacokinetics. In order for *in vitro* research on a medicinal plant to be relevant to herbal therapy, the following conditions must apply to the compound(s) responsible for the observed activity:

- It must be stable in the pharmaceutical preparation of the plant.
- It must not be changed by the digestive tract.
- It must be absorbed in significant quantities.
- It must survive its first passage through the liver.
- It must cross the blood-brain barrier (if relevant).
- It must be transported to the site of activity in significant quantities (based on the normal therapeutic dose and the concentration used in the *in vitro* study).
- It must not be inactivated by body fluids.
- It must gain access to the cell or receptor (if relevant).

(Obviously, many of these conditions would not apply if the plant preparation is used by topical application.)

Natural products are unlikely to fulfill all of these criteria. For example, they are often changed by digestive enzymes or bowel flora, and can be too large to be absorbed across the digestive tract. This does not necessarily detract from the therapeutic potential of medicinal plants, but rather serves to highlight the complexities of this field and the limitations of *in vitro* research.

It follows that the interpretation of *in vitro* research on plant extracts or isolated plant compounds is fraught with difficulties and uncertainties. Enthusiastic extrapolations of *in vitro* data result in misguided interpretations of how an herb might be used therapeutically or how it might act in the body. Such misinterpretations now abound in the herbal literature, presenting a major problem for those who are inexperienced or poorly trained. Such extrapolations are also often used to generate spurious concerns about toxicity or potential adverse reactions. (For a good example of this, see the many cautions and contraindications cited in Newall, C.A. et al, *Herbal Medicines, A Guide for Health-Care Professionals*, The Pharmaceutical Press, London (1996).) Many of the above reservations also apply to animal experiments, especially if the test dose is very high or is given by injection.

The media is quick to disseminate this kind of misinformation, and scientists often appear to be all too willing collaborators. This was well illustrated by a recent study where a team of scientists at Loma Linda University School of Medicine in California undertook studies to analyse the effects of some popular herbs on sperm DNA and on the fertilisation process.[2] Despite the wild claims made around this *in vitro* study, a careful analysis of the results revealed it did not uncover any real safety concerns.

Many pharmacological screening programs using *in vitro* tests on herbs, such as the program of the National Cancer Institute in the US, first remove "interfering" compounds like tannins. Tannins, which are common in herbs, can bind non-specifically to proteins such as enzymes, effectively producing false positive results. In addition, tannins have very low bioavailability, so any observed non-specific activity on intracellular enzymes is little more than a scientific curiosity. This consideration was well demonstrated by an elegant but perhaps ultimately futile study published recently in the *Journal of Ethnopharmacology*.[3] Owen and Johns found that the inhibitory activity of 26 plants on the enzyme xanthine oxidase was positively correlated with their tannin content ($p<0.001$).

The many and impressive *in vitro* pharmacological properties of tannins have little relevance to phytotherapy. For example *Epilobium parviflorum*, the small-flowered willow herb, was promoted 15 years ago by the Austrian herbalist Maria Treben as useful in the treatment of bladder and particularly prostate disorders, even cancer. More recently, P. Bohinsky, a Slovakian herbalist, briefly cited the benefits of other small species of Epilobium in benign prostate hyperplasia (BPH). To date, attempts to find the chemical components responsible for such activity have been largely unsuccessful. A team of French and Czech scientists decided to test the hypothesis that the biological effect of these herbs might be explained in terms of inhibition of 5-α-reductase, the enzyme responsible for the biosynthesis of dihydrotestosterone from testosterone.[4] Several extracts from *Epilobium parviflorum* were evaluated in an *in vitro* biochemical assay with 5-α-reductase. Only the aqueous extract showed significant inhibition of the enzyme, and the main active compound was identified as a macrocyclic tannin, oenothein B.

The study highlights some of the cautions cited above which need to be applied to the interpretation of *in vitro* research on medicinal plants. In this study, such considerations cast some doubt on the significance of the findings. Oenothein B is a large hydrolyzable tannin. Being a hydrolyzable tannin, it will probably be hydrolyzed (decomposed) by gastric acid. Even if it were not decomposed, oenothein B is too large to be absorbed into the bloodstream in significant quantities. Moreover, oenothein B is a tannin with 22 free phenolic groups. As such, it is likely to have a strong affinity for proteins and would demonstrate inhibition of most enzyme-based test models. In other words, the compound has non-specific activity, which considerably weakens the pharmacological significance of any positive findings.

The 5-α-reductase inhibitory potency of oenothein B was about 2000 times weaker than finasteride (Proscar), which is the reference compound for this class of inhibitors. This suggests that, in the unlikely event that oenothein B was transported to the prostate in significant quantities, it would still be unlikely to exert significant activity.

The concept of 5-α-reductase inhibition as a therapeutic strategy for BPH arose from biochemical speculation about the nature of this disorder. This model will not necessarily explain the therapeutic activity of plants used for BPH. For example, saw palmetto is considerably weaker than finasteride as an inhibitor of 5-α-reductase,[5] and yet has been found to be clinically superior to this compound in the management of BPH.[6] Although the authors of the above study on Epilobium have taken out a patent on their findings, their enthusiasm may be premature.

I have attended talks by herbalists or natural therapists who list many hypothetical activities for herbs derived from *in vitro* or *in vivo* research as if they were absolute facts. Moreover, they often fail to clarify in their presentations which information comes from pharmacological models and which has been proven in clinical trials. Extrapolation from pharmacological studies should be clearly stated and the information regarded as only of tentative relevance to a clinical situation.

Space precludes additional examples of misinformation, but there are many. As we move into a new millennium, information overload is almost overwhelming in our society. What many people earlier this century dreamed would be a new age of understanding and rationality has become to others a confusing nightmare. We are faced with a similar challenge and must be discerning with regard to the quality of information that is disseminated about herbal medicines.

The Challenge of Safety

Understanding the safety issues and demonstrating the safe use of herbal medicines is probably the biggest challenge which faces the future widespread use of medicinal plants. Already the media are carrying articles such as the examples above that only serve to frighten the public away from what might be a valuable therapeutic option.

There is no doubt that a considerable bias exists in the media on the reporting of safety issues concerning herbs. The following brief article appeared on page 2 of the Brisbane (Australia) *Courier-Mail* on Wednesday, May 15, 1996:

Fatal Curatives

More than 100 deaths from liver problems had been linked to 13 antibiotics and other drugs used between 1972 and March 1996, the Adverse Drug Reactions Advisory Committee said yesterday. The committee said that although *some* of the 13 drugs could save lives, *doctors should take care in prescribing them.*

This understated article is extraordinary in many respects, including the title. In particular, naturopaths and phytotherapists may be surprised at the committee's mild response to drugs that are consistently causing loss of life due to hepatotoxicity. By contrast, based on only the slightest association of hepatotoxicity, several countries have completely banned the use of several herbs, such as comfrey, coltsfoot, and hemp agrimony.

When it comes to concerns about safety, why are herbs treated so differently from drugs? The same article would have elicited horrified headlines if it had been about herbal medicines. This is a complex issue with many aspects. By contrast, the German government, for example, takes the attitude that presumes herbs, being natural medicines, to be completely safe. Hence, even the slightest doubt about safety is unacceptable. But is it reasonable to expect absolute safety for medicinal plants?

The safety of a medicine can never be considered in isolation from its efficacy. This is known as risk-benefit assessment. Such an assessment is qualitative, not quantitative (in other words, the division of a number for risk by a number for efficacy is never actually performed), and hence always involves some element of subjectivity. For example, a greater safety risk is acceptable when a life-saving drug is used to save a life than when used for other purposes. This is the reason dangerous therapeutic drugs are tolerated by the regulators and perhaps explains the mild response of the committee quoted in the newspaper article above.

A major problem in the assessment of many herbal medicines is the lack of hard data supporting their efficacy. If the authorities eye their benefit to be zero, any risk at all becomes unacceptable. One positive development in this area could be the acceptance of well-established traditional use as evidence for efficacy. Nonetheless, the fact remains that in order to protect the status of herbal medicines, information is required about efficacy as well as safety.

The safety issues facing herbal medicine are often distorted by the scientific community. Imagine that tea were a newly introduced herb. Tea is the dried fermented leaves of *Camellia sinensis*, an herb indigenous to the Indian sub-continent. Tea contains caffeine and tannins as its main consituents.[7] A superficial examination of the literature reveals the following: caffeine is a known teratogen,[8] a suspected carcinogen,[9] and in animal feeding studies causes severe weight loss and thymic and testicular atrophy.[10] Tannins have demonstrated carcinogenic effects; they inhibit digestive enzymes, inhibit mineral absorption and are highly toxic to the liver and kidneys.[11] Human deaths have resulted from the administration of tannic acid.[12] The carcinogenic activity[13] and toxicity[14] of the tannins from tea have been demonstrated in animal experiments. In human studies tea can cause thiamin deficiency[15] and constipation.[16] Epidemiological studies have linked black tea consumption with rectal[17] and esophageal cancers.[13] Of course, common sense tells us normal use of tea is safe (probably even beneficial, as recent research is showing) but the scientific information taken out of context is quite damning, in fact more alarming than that for commonly used herbs.

It is worthwhile to examine why this considerable scientific evidence for the "toxic nature of tea" has not made headlines and has not resulted in tea being restricted or entirely banned in the public interest. Just as a series of promising pharmacological studies does not imply the birth of a new wonder drug, the findings of toxicological studies can be of only minor relevance to the common experience. Differences such as species studied, interaction with nutrients, dose, form and duration of dose, all combine to explain why the results for tea and its components would have little bearing on the moderate consumption of the beverage. Phytotherapists should therefore be forgiven for taking a similar stance about herbs. The main difference is that toxicologists and legislators are familiar with tea, but see herbs as alien and unnecessary, so they are prepared to believe the worst. How much credibility would a scientist have if she raised sensationalist concerns in the media about the safety of tea? Yet scientists do the same thing for commonly used herbs.

The safe use of herbal medicines during pregnancy is becoming an increasingly contentious issue. On the one hand, some regulatory authorities advocate the policy that if there is no clear evidence of safety from controlled clinical trials, then an herb should not be recommended during pregnancy. This was well illustrated by some recent deliberations of the Complementary Medicines Evaluation Committee (CMEC) of the Australian Therapeutic Goods Administration (equivalent to America's FDA). CMEC was assessing the safe use of over-the-counter products containing kava (*Piper methysticum*) and came to the conclusion, despite the lack of evidence for harm from kava during pregnancy, that kava products should carry the following warning: "Not for prolonged use. If symptoms persist seek advice from a health care practitioner. Those who are pregnant or nursing are not recommended to use Kava."

If this restriction were applied to all commonly used herbs, then probably only ginger, senna, and ginseng would be exempted from such a warning. Ironically, some herbal and scientific authors believe that these three herbs are contraindicated in pregnancy.

Yet some scientists with little clinical experience in the use of herbs have speculated about harmful effects that might ensue from the use of herbs during pregnancy. They appear to adopt the stance that even if a negative effect from an herb is only remotely possible (highly unlikely), then that herb should not be taken during pregnancy. The unspoken assumption here is that herbs are only marginally efficacious, if at all, so even the remotest risk during pregnancy is unacceptable. This approach is exemplified by the list provided in the book by Newall and co-authors.[18] According to these authors, many innocuous herbs are contraindicated in pregnancy. Their conclusions are largely based on extrapolations from pharmacological studies on plants or isolated plant constituents.

Even herbalists are willing to speculate. In *Herb Contraindications and Drug Interactions*, Francis Brinker suggests that the following relatively innocuous herbs are unsafe to take during pregnancy: alfalfa, lemon balm, basil, black pepper, burdock, calendula, catnip, chamomile, dill, fennel, fenugreek, flaxseed, garlic, gotu kola, lavender, licorice, passionflower, rosemary, and St John's Wort.[19] Ironically, many of these herbs are enjoyed as foods, teas, or spices by the general populace, including pregnant women. How is it that an herb which is regarded as completely safe by herbalists, the general public, and regulatory authorities, suddenly becomes so dangerous when a woman is pregnant?

So essentially, the list of herbs safe to take during pregnancy is determined by the stance which is taken. If the requirement is for evidence of safety from controlled clinical trials in pregnant women, then that list is very short. If a speculative approach is taken, then no herbs should be taken during pregnancy, because it is very likely that every plant will contain some compound which, given in massive doses under highly artificial conditions, would show some effect which could be construed to be detrimental during pregnancy. To be consistent, no plant foods would be taken during pregnancy as well. This is clearly a nonsensical extreme.

We clearly need more information on the safety of herbs. Since they are already being used every day by millions of people worldwide, the most sensible and ethical approach is to observe those people already taking herbs. Such observational studies will provide information about toxicity, herb-drug interactions, adverse reactions and reproductive safety. The funding of such studies should be an urgent priority for governments.

Most countries of the world have a system of adverse reaction reporting. Such systems are rarely used by traditional practitioners, herbalists, or naturopaths. There is clearly a need to extend these reporting systems to the people who prescribe herbs the most. There are several weaknesses in relying on medical practitioners as the main profession to report adverse reactions to herbal medicines.

I once received a phone call from a nearby hospital. A young doctor was inquiring about my herbal treatment of a patient who had been admitted with pronounced jaundice. The doctor stated that the patient had elevated serum liver enzymes consistent with an adverse drug reaction, and my prescribed herbal liquid formula was a prime suspect. I tried to assure the doctor that the formula, which contained an Echinacea root blend, meadowsweet, and chamomile, could not be responsible for such a severe reaction. I also pointed out that the patient had been taking this formula for many months without any problem. The doctor was not reassured, and confidently stated that he knew of a few cases of hepatotoxicity caused by Echinacea. When questioned, the doctor admitted that the information came from a gastroenterologist, and that he had not actually seen or read about such reactions from Echinacea. Moreover, he conceded that the patient's condition could also be due to an infection, though his limited tests were negative. Further investigation revealed that the patient worked in a veterinary laboratory and was potentially exposed to exotic viral infections. He had also been working long hours and was run down. Just before the jaundice developed, the patient had symptoms consistent with a viral infection, such as fever and malaise, but the hospital had not extensively tested for viruses. Despite the more likely conclusion that jaundice was caused by an unusual viral infection, the patient never returned for further herbal treatment. It is disconcerting that patients sometimes accept the less-informed judgments of allopathic doctors over those of their phytotherapists.

Are herbs a likely cause of hepatotoxicity and other adverse reactions, as has been proposed by some literature? Only a rational and objective approach, with careful collection and analysis of case histories, will properly answer this question. Objective evaluation by the medical profession is not likely to occur in the current political climate. Most doctors have received no training in herbal medicine and are hostile towards or dismissive of its therapeutic value and safety. In such an environment of bias, the finger is pointed at the herbal treatment as if to say: "I told you so." Coincidences do occur, and unknown causes can operate. If these factors are not taken into account, the "dangers" of herbal medicine will certainly become a self-fulfilling prophecy. The subject of herb-drug interactions requires much more study, both at experimental and observational levels.

The uncertainties created by the lack of objective information about herbal safety, coupled with the growing tendencies to make increasingly potent preparations of herbs in conveniently smaller forms with the use of concentrated extracts, tempt governments to impose restrictive regulations on the future development of phytotherapy.

Herbal products can be regulated either as dietary supplements (foods) or therapeutics (medicines). Depending on the relevant legislation in each country, manufacturers can choose to position their products in the marketplace as either foods or medicines. In some parts of the world, as appears to be the case in Europe, the food option is being closed off, while the bar to register a medicine is way too high. This could soon lead to a situation in the UK where tinctures prescribed by herbalists and the majority of herbal products sold in health food stores will become illegal.

Even in countries such as the U.S., where herbs are sold as dietary supplements, the threat of over-regulation exists. The Codex is an attempt to harmonize international food standards in order to remove regulatory barriers to free trade. But it is possible that the bureaucratic net created by the adoption of this agreement could result in the restriction of some herbs. It is important that governments listen to consumers when legislating control of herbal products. Consumers want the ready availability of safe and effective herbal products. Only a foolhardy government would seek to unnecessarily restrict this flow.

The Challenge of Quality

Herbs are sourced from nature and hence, unlike conventional chemical drugs, vary from batch to batch. This can be readily understood by comparison with another plant product: wine. In technical terms, wine is the fermented juice of the fruit of *Vitis vinifera*. However, factors such as the grape variety, climatic conditions, soil type, time of harvest and fermentation conditions can all determine whether a batch of wine will be either poor or good quality (as subsequently reflected in the price of the wine!).

In the case of wine, measures such as the texture, color, aroma, and taste determine if the product is of good quality or otherwise. For medicinal plants, the situation is much more complex. Most of the chemical components of herbs important for therapeutic activity are secondary metabolites. By definition, secondary metabolites are not thought to be important for the growth and survival of the plant, although they are sometimes produced in higher levels in response to infection, insect attack, or adverse growing conditions.

One consequence of this is that even though they may give an impression of quality, the appearance and color of an herb are not necessarily indicators of its therapeutic quality. Indeed, plants grown under adverse conditions may sometimes have a poor appearance but higher levels of secondary metabolites. A corollary of this is that while herb batches that have a good appearance and a pleasant taste might be suitable for herbal teas, they may not be optimal for use as medicines.

An example is chamomile. Chamazulene is considered to be an important active component, and varieties of chamomile have been bred which have higher levels of its precursor compound matricine. Since matricine imparts a bitter taste to the flowers, these high medicinal grade varieties are not suitable for an herbal tea taken for pleasure.

How can the quality of an herb be determined? One approach adopted by the various pharmacopoeias and used by manufacturers is to set minimum levels of marker chemical compounds for an herbal raw material. These are seen to give an indication of activity, and hence quality. (This approach is fraught with difficulties. Even where the marker compound is known to contribute to the therapeutic activity of the herb—and this is not always the case—phytotherapists stress that the chemical complexity of the plant confers the sum total of its activity.) Until we better understand how individual herbs work in their chemical totality, it is a good starting point. The uncertainties can be lessened by choosing phytochemical classes of marker compounds (flavonoids, essential oils, oligomeric procyanidins, etc.) rather than just individual chemical components. In addition, testing for plural marker compounds (or groups of marker compounds) in the same plant can lead to a better assessment of activity. As one researcher recently commented: "If a batch of an herb contains low levels of one marker compound, and then by a completely different test also shows low levels of another class of marker compound, we can begin to form the conclusion that it is of poor quality." Yet we need considerably more information about how the various components in an herb interact to confer therapeutic efficacy. This will in turn impact on assessments of quality.

There is a much simpler quality issue that plagues herbal medicine, the issue of adulteration. Perhaps the most commonly documented reason for adverse reactions to herbal medicines is the presence of adulterants. This adulteration may be due to:

- Environmental contamination of the herb with a chemical or pathogen.
- Unintentional substitution of one or more herbal ingredients with a toxic species.
- Intentional addition of a "natural" active component which is responsible for the adverse reaction, such as a microorganism, mineral or nutrient.
- Intentional addition of a conventional chemical drug, either of natural or synthetic origin.

These problems can generally be overcome by responsible manufacture, adequate testing, and above all, commitment to pharmaceutical-level Good Manufacturing Practice (GMP).

Examples of these four types of adulteration have appeared in the recent scientific literature. A report from Taiwan describes a case study of a patient who developed a unique syndrome of multiple renal tubular dysfunction after ingestion of a Chinese herbal formula contaminated by cadmium.[20]

A letter to the *British Medical Journal* in 1996 asserted that Podophyllum poisoning has developed into a mini-epidemic in Hong Kong.[21] The poisoning is caused by ingestion of the herb known in Cantonese as Gwai-Kou, derived from the roots and rhizomes of *Podophyllum hexandrum* (also known as *P. emodi*). The herb appeared in Hong Kong in 1989 as an adulterant of Lung-Dam-Cho (*Gentiana spp.*) and led to two cases of neuropathy and encephalopathy. Around the same period, this herb was found in Taipei and Kuala Lumpur as an adulterant of another herb, Wai-Ling-Sin, which is the root of *Clematis spp.* Recently, nine cases of neuropathy have been reported in Hong Kong. About 10 percent of 234 samples of Wai-Ling-Sin taken from Hong Kong outlets were found to be Podophyllum!

Sometimes unintentional adulteration can occur when harvesting an herb from the wild for personal use. Veno-occlusive disease of the liver was diagnosed in an 18-month-old boy who had regularly consumed an herbal tea mixture.[22] The tea contained peppermint and what the mother thought was coltsfoot (*Tussilago farfara*). However, macroscopic and microscopic analysis of the leaf material indicted that the parents had mistakenly gathered alpendost (*Adenostyles alliariae*) instead of coltsfoot. The two plants can be confused, especially after the flowering period. This may also explain why coltsfoot has developed a reputation as a toxic herb in some quarters.

Perhaps the worst and most tragic example of herbal adulteration in the western world occurred in Belgium, where a group of medical doctors running a slimming program included some herbs in their treatment. One of the herbs they wished to include was *Stephania tetrandra,* but patients in fact received *Aristolochia fangchi* which contains aristolochic acid.[23,24] This substitution is relatively common. The women were also taking acetazolamide, a sulfonamide drug which can cause metabolic acidosis, anorexia and weight loss and can also be nephrotoxic. Many women suffered severe kidney damage. The acetazolamide potentiated the nephrotoxicity of the herbal aristolochic acid by decreasing acidification (i.e., increasing pH) in renal tissue. Two women involved in this tragedy have subsequently developed urothelial cancer due to the genotoxicity of aristolochic acid.[25] Careful attention needs to be paid to prevent such dangers of drug interactions.

The Challenge of Disease Prevention

Since they normally show low toxicity and are consumed on a regular basis as foods and beverages, herbs are ideally suited as preventative treatments. This could prove to be their greatest therapeutic value. In this context, proof of safety and efficacy is paramount, since the effort, expense, and potential risks of taking a treatment over a long period of time are considerable. This is precisely why many pharmaceuticals are proving to be problematical as preventative agents.

How can information about disease prevention by herbs be obtained? One way is epidemiological studies. This can be illustrated by the influence of ginseng consumption on cancer.[26,27] Another example is garlic consumption and cancer. Eleven epidemiological studies in six countries have demonstrated a correlation between garlic consumption and decreased risk of gastrointestinal (particularly stomach and colon) cancers and breast and endometrial cancer.[28]

A French research team has been investigating the effects of various factors including alcohol consumption on the risk of developing dementia and Alzheimer's disease (AD).[29] Their prospective study (looking forward) began in 1988 on a group of 3777 men and women over 65 years of age living in or near Bordeaux. As might be expected, wine was almost the only form of alcohol consumed.

Three years after beginning the study, 99 of the 2273 people left in the group had dementia, including 66 with AD. The researchers found, perhaps to their surprise, that mild to moderate wine consumption appeared to significantly protect against senile dementia and AD. After adjustment for various confounding factors, mild drinkers (up to 2 glasses of wine a day) had a 55 percent ($p<0.05$) chance of developing AD compared to non-drinkers, and for moderate drinkers (2 to 4 glasses a day) the relative risk was only 28 percent ($p<0.05$). Significant protection was not observed for heavy drinkers (more than 5 glasses a day).

Taking dementia as a whole (including AD), only moderate drinkers exhibited a significantly reduced risk of developing dementia compared to non-drinkers (19 percent, $p<0.01$). Mortality rates were also significantly lower among mild and moderate drinkers.

Why should wine have this protective effect against dementia? Topping the list of possible reasons are the antioxidant components of wine, particularly the oligomeric procyanidins (OPC) and resveratrol in red wine. It is interesting therefore to speculate that grape seed extract (*Vitis vinifera*) might have similar protective properties. Thus the epidemiological data on red wine consumption could provide valuable leads about the diseases which OPC (in the form of grape seed or hawthorn extract) and resveratrol (as extracts of certain Chinese *Polygonum species*) might prevent.

The Challenge of the Patient

The use of herbs is part of a therapeutic system—good phytotherapy is not just about substituting a plant medicine for a chemical medicine. A one-dimensional model of herbal practice, using herbs just like drugs, is not an intelligent role for phytotherapy in the next millennium.

Used properly and in context, good science has much to offer phytotherapy. But what is the proper context? In particular, scientific investigation is useful for providing the solid, factual, background information that any therapist needs. For example, science can tell us that *Ginkgo biloba* is good for circulation or that *Hypericum perforatum* is a valid treatment for depression. However, traditional considerations will often be more relevant in guiding the phytotherapist as to when to apply this information in a clinical situation. In this context, science is just one tool to be used in the consulting room. During a consultation, a good practitioner will assess the patient as an individual using careful observation, listening, insight, logic, and common sense, supported by the appropriate use of scientific information. The treatment of the patient as an individual can never be outweighed by results of double-blind clinical trials.

In any examination of the worth and future potential of herbal medicines, their traditional therapeutic context should not be discarded. To do so will limit the value of herbs and make them subservient to modern reductionist thinking and superficial symptom control. In a landmark study published in *JAMA*, a team of Australian scientists examined the effect of traditional Chinese medicines in the treatment of irritable bowel syndrome. Under double-blind conditions one group of patients received a standard formula, another were given a placebo, and a third group received an individual formulation prescribed after a traditional consultation. Results from the individual treatment and the standard formula were similar and demonstrated a significant benefit for both treatment groups above placebo. So at first glance it would appear that this study found no advantage for individual treatment above a preconceived formula. However, follow-up investigation found that the patients who received individual treatment experienced better long-term results.[30]

My main herbal teacher, Hein Zeylstra, cautioned me as follows:

> Everyone is at a loss to keep up with the flow from the scientific press, and before the bewildered 'herbalists' realize what is going on, their domain is stolen from under their feet by the scientific world. Scientific congresses on phytotherapy are popping up all over the world, in some countries every two to three years, blasting the newfound treasures to the astonished audiences.
>
> That is what the scene is about now, and where is the herbalist going? The new phytotherapist steps in. What is his or her role? First of all, the phytotherapist should not throw the baby away with the bath water. The herbalist had and still has many valuables. At least there is some form of philosophy, consisting of a bit of old European tradition and physio-medicalism. Of course most of the traditional medicines have a philosophy or rather a system, a kind of guide for the application of herbs. Modern medicine and modern pharmacology have no philosophy at all. Moreover, herbalists are usually trying to deal with underlying causes instead of suppressing symptoms....

Ever since my training as a medical herbalist, I have maintained a particular interest in the cause and treatment of diseases that do not arise from a single cause. In fact, it is quite possible that the same diseases will have different causes from person to person. The current approach in medical science is not very comfortable with such an idea. However, traditionally-based systems of medicine such as phytotherapy place great emphasis on the treatment of the individual. What we need is a multi-factorial model which allows us to individualize treatments, yet at the same time takes into account the most likely factors operating in each particular case. This requires a blend of traditional understanding with the latest research findings. Such a synthesis is the goal of the modern phytotherapist.

The Challenge of Sustainability

Until a few years ago, I was using *Pygeum africanum* for the treatment of benign prostatic hyperplasia and found it a very effective medicine. However, I stopped using this herb when *Pygeum* gained endangered status, entirely due to over-harvesting of wild stands in Africa caused by the strong demand for this herb in France. Other alternatives such as saw palmetto were available. It is the duty and responsibility of herbal companies and practitioners to ensure that the promotion and use of any herb does not endanger its existence.

This situation applies in many countries. The wildcrafted herbs golden seal (*Hydrastis canadensis*), false unicorn (*Helonias luteum*) and *Echinacea angustifolia* root, all from the USA, are becoming increasingly more expensive and difficult to obtain. While golden seal now has endangered status and false unicorn is nearing endangered status, there is developing evidence that this status also could apply to *Echinacea angustifolia*, and its harvesting is now being restricted in several states. Fortunately for Echinacea users, cultivated *E. purpurea* root is readily available, and cultivated *E. angustifolia* root is becoming increasingly so. Nonetheless, the price of *E. angustifolia* will continue to rise until such time that large quantities are available from growers.

American herbalists have supported the initiative to develop an organization called United Plant Savers (UPS) in the USA. Their objectives are:

- Identifying the at-risk medicinal plants species.
- Researching cultivation and propagation techniques of at-risk medicinal plants.
- Securing and operating botanical sanctuaries, places to learn about at-risk medicinals, places to act as seed and plant material repositories, and places to carry on research into sustainable cultivation techniques.
- Replanting and restoring at-risk medicinal plants by grass roots efforts.
- Consulting with people growing and harvesting medicinal herbs regarding sustainable land practices.

- Raising public awareness of the current plight of threatened medicinal herbs.
- Working with the natural products industry to bring awareness to all concerned.

UPS has developed an "At Risk" list and a "Watch" list. While some details of these lists are controversial, their work is generally to be commended.

Another organization working in this field is Europe's TRAFFIC. Recently the first International Symposium on the Conservation of Medicinal Plants in Trade in Europe was organized by TRAFFIC Europe. According to trade surveys undertaken in eight different European countries, and summarized in a recent TRAFFIC publication (Europe's Medicinal and Aromatic Plants: Their Use, Trade and Conservation), at least 150 medicinal and aromatic plant species are threatened as a result of over-collection, destructive harvesting techniques, habitat loss and habitat changes, in one or several European countries of their area of distribution. The report detailed the following species as endangered: *Adonis vernalis, Arctostaphylos uva-ursi, Arnica montana, Cetraria islandica, Drosera rotundifolia, Gentiana lutea, Glycyrrhiza glabra, Gypsophila* spp.*, Ankyropetalum gypsophylloides, Menyanthes trifoliata,* species of Orchidaceae that are used in the production of salep, *Paeonia* spp., *Primula* spp., *Ruscus aculeatus* and *Sideritis* spp. Two of these taxa, namely *Arnica montana* and *Drosera* spp. were the subject of specific talks at the symposium. Of course, many endangered or at risk species are now available from cultivated sources, and it is vital that such procurement be encouraged.

We have seen that there are many challenges facing phytotherapy today; and we have also noted that there are intelligent ways to respond to each of these challenges. With the goodwill and cooperation of governments, media, our medical colleagues, and the general public, phytotherapists can render cost-effective health services in natural and sustainable ways: building upon the long traditions of herbal wisdom in the cultures of the world, and adapting their research and practices to the needs of modern patients.

Notes

1. Keplinger, K., Laus, G., Wurm, M. et al., "*Uncaria tomentosa* (Willd. DC)—Ethnomedicinal use and new pharmacological, toxicological and botanical results." *Journal of Ethnopharmacology* 1999, 64: 23-24.

2. Ondrizek, R. R., Chan, P. J., Patton, W. C. et al., "An alternative medicine study of herbal effects on the penetration of zona-free hamster oocytes and the integrity of sperm deoxyribonucleic acid." *Fertil. Steril.* 1999, 71: 517-522. (See my review of this study in *The Townsend Letter for Doctors and Patients,* June, 1999).

3. Owen, P. L., Johns, T., "Xanthine oxidase inhibitory activity of northeastern North American plant remedies used for gout." *Journal of Ethnopharmacology*, 1999, 64: 149-160.

4. Lessuisse, D., Berjonneau, J., Ciot, C. et al., "Determination of oenothein B as the active 5-alpha-reductase-inhibiting principle of the folk medicine *Epilobium parviflorum*." *J Nat Prod* 1996, 59 (5): 490-492.

5. Rhodes, L., Primka, R. L., Berman, C. et al., "Comparison of finasteride (Proscar), a 5-alpha reductase inhibitor, and various commercial plant extracts in *in vitro* and *in vivo* 5-alpha reductase inhibition." *Prostate,* 1993, 22 (1): 43-51.

6. Bach, D. "Treatment of the benign prostate hypertrophy." *Phytopathologische Zeitschrift,* 1996, 17 (4): 209-212, 215-218.

7. Trease, G. E., Evans, W. C., *Pharmacognosy, 12th ed.* London: Balliere Tindall, 1983, p. 622.

8. Collins, T. F., Welsh, J. J., Black, T. N. et al., "Potential reversibility of skeletal effects in rats exposed *in utero* to caffeine." *Food Chem Toxicol.* 1987, 25 (9): 647-662.

9. Rosenkranz, H. S., Ennever, F. K., "Evaluation of the genotoxicity of theobromine and caffeine." *Food Chem Toxicol.* 1987, 25 (3): 247-251.

10. Gans, J. H., "Comparative toxicities of dietary caffeine and theobromine in the rat." *Food Chem Toxicol.* 1984, 22 (5): 365-369.

11. Deshpande, S. S,, Sathe, S.K., Salunkhe, D.K., "Chemistry and safety of

plant polyphenols." *Adv Exp Med Biol.* 1984, 177: 457-495.

12. Krezanoski, J. Z., "Tannic acid: chemistry, analysis, and toxicology – An episode in the pharmaceutics of radiology." *Radiology,* 1966, 87 (4): 655-7.

13. Morton, J. F., "Tea with milk." *Science,* 1979, 204 (4396): 909.

14. Panda, N. C., Sahu, B. K., Panda, S. K. et al., "Damage done to intestine, liver and kidneys by tannic acid of tea and coffee." *Indian J Nutr and Diet* 1981: 18 (3): 97-103.

15. Ruenwongsa, P., Pattanavibag, S., "Effect of tea consumption on the levels of alpha-ketoglutarate and pyruvate dehydrogenase in rat brain." *Experientia,* 1982, 38 (7): 787-788.

16. Hojgaard, L., Arffmann, S., Jorgensen, M. et al., "Tea consumption: a cause of constipation?" *BMJ. (Clin Res Ed.)* 1981, 282 (6267): 864.

17. Heilbrun, L. K., Nomura, A., Stemmermann, G. N., "Black tea consumption and cancer risk: a prospective study." *Br J Cancer,* 1986, 54 (4): 677-683.

18. Newall, C. A., Anderson, L. A., Phillipson, J. D., *Herbal Medicines, A Guide for Health-Care Professionals.* London: Pharmaceutical Press, 1996.

19. Brinker, F., *Herb Contraindications and Drug Interactions.* Sandy, Oregon: Eclectic Institute, 1997.

20. Wu, M. S., Hong, J. J., Lin, J. L. et al., "Multiple tubular dysfunction induced by mixed Chinese herbal medicines containing cadmium." *Nephrol Dial Transplant,* 1996, 11 (5): 867-870.

21. But, P. P., Tomlinson, B., Cheung, K. O. et al., "Adulterants of herbal products can cause poisoning." *BMJ.* 1996, 313 (7049): 117.

22. Sperl, W., Stuppner, H., Gassner, I. et al., "Reversible hepatic veno-occlusive disease in an infant after consumption of pyrrolizidine-containing herbal tea." *Eur J Pediatr.* 1995, 154 (2): 112-116.

23. Vanherweghem, J. L., Depierreux, M., Tielemans, C. et al., "Rapidly progressive interstitial renal fibrosis in young women: association with slimming regimen including Chinese herbs." *Lancet,* 1993, 341 (8842): 387-391.

24. Vanhaelen, M., Vanhaelen-Fastre, R., But, P. et al., "Identification of aristolochic acid in Chinese herbs." *Lancet,* 1994, 343 (8890): 174.

25. Reginster, F., Jadoul, M., van Ypersele de Strihou, C., "Chinese herbs nephropathy presentation, natural history and fate after transplantation." *Nephrol Dial Transplant.* 1997, 12 (1): 81-86.

26. Yun, T. K., Choi, S. Y., "A case-control study of ginseng intake and cancer." *Int J Epidemiol.* 1990, 19 (4): 871-876.

27. Yun, T. K., Choi, S. Y., "Preventive effect of ginseng intake against various human cancers: a case-control study on 1987 pairs." *Cancer Epidemiol Biomarkers Prev.* 1995, 4 (4): 401-408. (See my review of this work in *The Townsend Letter for Doctors and Patients,* October, 1999.)

28. Lawson, L. D. "Garlic: A review of its medicinal effects and indicated active compounds." In: Lawson, L. D., & Bauer, R. (eds). *Phytomedicines of Europe: Chemistry and Biological Activity.* ACS Symposium Series 691. Washington DC: American Chemical Society, 1998, pp. 176-209.

29. Orgogozo, J. M., Dartigues, J. F., Lafont, S. et al., "Wine consumption and dementia in the elderly: a prospective community study in the Bordeaux area." *Rev Neurol.* (Paris), 1997, 153 (3): 185-192.

30. Bensoussan, A., Talley, N. J., Hing, M. et al., "Treatment of irritable bowel syndrome with Chinese herbal medicine." *JAMA.* 1998, 280 (18): 1585-1589.

The Body as a Barometer of the Mind

10.

Comprehensive Medicine
Its Philosophy and Methodology

Katsutaro Nagata M.D., Ph.D.
Hamamatsu University School of Medicine, Japan

Introduction: On Quality Medical Care

Modern medicine is now facing a great crisis. "Comprehensive Medicine" can solve these problems by improving medical treatment to make it more complete. This medicine takes the viewpoint that a patient should be treated as an "individual person suffering from an illness." "Individual person" here indicates a whole person or a "bio-psycho-socio-existential integrity." This is the essential nature of medicine. To our regret, modern medicine alone can never achieve complete treatment. Comprehensive medicine should not be merely an imaginary one; it should be utilized effectively. The practice of comprehensive medicine for patients "suffering here and now" by making best use of currently available medical resources (both personal and material) should be established systemically. For this purpose, we should recognize both the indications and limitations of modern Western medicine, and then incorporate traditional Oriental medicine and psychosomatic medicine to integrate these three medicines on the basis of good research. In clinical practice, we should establish doctor-patient relationships with deep mutual respect on the basis of wide knowledge and deep wisdom as experts, and also should have the sensitivity to differentiate the use of science from that of art.

In developed countries today, quantitatively effective medical treatments are available, but qualitatively, patients are far from satisfied. Comprehensive medicine can be proffered as a system of medicine which ensures both quantitative and qualitative satisfaction (Day, 1980). Comprehensive medicine understands patients holistically as "suffering persons." The purpose of comprehensive medicine is to provide well-balanced medical treatment efficiently so as to ensure patients a higher quality of life. Comprehensive medicine represents a growing trend in the modern world.

What is comprehensive medicine? Comprehensive medicine emphasizes not the correction of symptoms alone but rather treats patients as "whole persons suffering from illness," understanding them from a bio-psycho-socio-existential viewpoint. To reach this understanding, comprehensive medicine tries to solve problems specific to individual patients. This tendency responds to the social demand that medicine improve qualitatively. Concretely, comprehensive medicine aims at improving patients' QOL, respecting the characteristics of individual patients. The practice of comprehensive medicine should:

1) Respect individuality of each patient, maintaining balance between cure and care.
2) Guarantee quality as well as quantity of medical treatment.
3) Try to improve Quality of Life (QOL) according to the circumstances of each patient.
4) Improve both therapeutic and economic efficiency of medical treatment.
5) Be teachable and commumicable, not depending on charismatic or intuitive personal skills.
6) Be assessable and carefully evaluated.

Comprehensive medicine comprehends patients as whole persons on a bio-psycho-socio-existential model, and emphasizes the importance of doctor-patient relationships to the healing process. Comprehensive medicine takes modern medicine as its base, adds traditional/Oriental medical approaches, and uses psychosomatic medicine as an interface bridging these two systems with mutual respect. Doctors should recognize the indications and limitations of each of these systems, tailoring them systematically and rationally to individual patients. Comprehensive medicine is an analytic and systematic as well as comprehensive science. In practicing comprehensive medicine, we should remain well aware of the indications and limitations of these three systems.

Cathartic Emergency Medicine and Complementary Preventive Maintenance

Modern Western medicine is strong in cathartic methods (Japanese: *Shahou*) including operations, chemotherapy, radiotherapy, and pharmaceuticals to suppress physical reactions, while traditional Oriental and psychosomatic medicine are strong in complementary methods (Japanese: *Hohou*) to avoid physical reactions. These systems are by no means mutually exclusive. As a specialist, a doctor should decide which method to employ on the basis of understanding the whole patient, guiding patients to maintain their overall balance. (Table 1 on the following page illustrates the differences of the two methodologies.)

The Role of Psychosomatic Medicine

The base of comprehensive medicine is understanding patients as whole persons from a psychosomatic viewpoint, based on Michael Balint's techniques of comprehensive medical interviews about the patients' bio-psycho-social problems (Balint, 1957). Through this method, doctors accept their patients as complex persons, supporting and reassuring them, reflecting the doctors' philosophy, views of living and dying, of medicine, of health and humanity. This is what Watkins (1978) calls cultivation of the "therapeutic self" in medical education; a comprehensive medical education should include not only certification of technical skills and qualifications,

Table 1: Cathartic and Complementary Approaches

	Cathartic Approach	Complementary Approach
Assessment	Current Western Methods	17-KS-S, QOL questionnaire
Bodily Function	To Control total/partial excesses by:	To Control total/partial excesses by:
Methods	Psychological Catharsis	Psychological analysis/counseling
	Surgical resection/exsanguination	Supplement deficiency (total or partial)
	Anticancer drugs and radiotherapy to kill cancerous cells	I.V.H., D.I., blood transfusions
	Antibiotics to kill bacteria	Endocrinological therapy (insulin, etc.)
	Anti-inflammatories to stop inflammation	Complementary drugs:
	Block pain (ß-blocker, H2 blocker, etc.)	Oriental herbal formulae (*Juzentaihotou*, Red ginseng, vitamins, Coenzyme Q10)
Background	Chiefly current Western medicine	Traditional Oriental/Psychosomatic medicine

(Nagata, K. V1, 1996)

but the training of each doctor's therapeutic attitude.

In actually carrying out comprehensive medicine, "care" must complement "cure," showing respect for patients' self control. "Cure" and "care" are like two wheels of a cart. At this point, philosophy, methodology and practice of comprehensive medicine are required. Table 2 shows the differences between them.

Progression of Disease Through Three Phases

Every illness progresses through three phases, viz.: health (the original/normal state) → functional disease (phase I) → organized disease (phase II) → fatal disease (phase III) → death.

The length (span) and quality of life (QOL) are greatly affected

Table 2: A Typology of Cure and Care

	CURE	CARE
Subjects	Diseased visceral organs and cells	Whole person suffering from disease
Basic character	Universal, analytic, scientific	Individual, integrative, humanist
Basic medical model	Acute disease model	Chronic disease model
	Anatomy (corpus model)	Comprehensive medical model
	Physiology (experimental animal model)	(Bio-psycho-socio-existential model)
Methodology	Analytical	Integrative of findings of analysis
	Morphological (diagnostic imaging)	Phenomenological
	Statistical	Personal experiential (interviews)
Objective	Cure of diseased visceral organs/cells	Improvement in QOL
Problem location	Patient's diseased visceral organs/cells	Both patients and relationships
Doctor-patient Relationship	Active-passive, or	Mutual participation
	Directive-cooperative Paternalism	Mutual respect (of patients and relationships)
Medical Education	Of knowledge and techniques (skills)	Of attitude and interrelationships (wisdom)
Evaluation	Quantitative, statistical, biochemical	Qualitative, personal, psycho-social

(Nagata, K., V3, 1997)

by genetic constitution, lifestyle, aging, stress, and coping styles. To maintain health, it is of primary importance to become aware of functional disease. Rescuing patients from alexithymia (loss of emotion), alexisomia (loss of sensation), and loss of meaning are matters of highest priority (see Figure 1 on following page).

Modern Western medicine is indicated for diagnosis and treatment of organized disease (phase II). (Japan's National Health Insurance system insures only such medical treatments.) However, Western medicine has little or no methodology for "unorganized" or functional disease. When laboratory tests detect no abnormalities, functional disease is written off as "psychosomatic," "all in the patient's mind," or "requiring further observation without

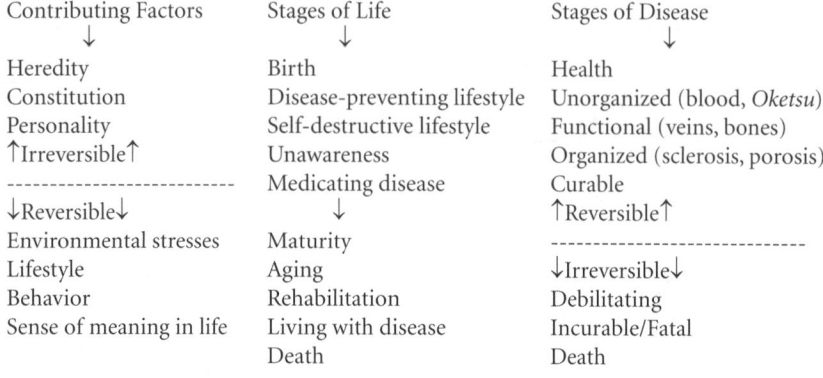

Figure 1. Progression of disease as seen from Comprehensive Medicine

Contributing Factors ↓	Stages of Life ↓	Stages of Disease ↓
Heredity	Birth	Health
Constitution	Disease-preventing lifestyle	Unorganized (blood, *Oketsu*)
Personality	Self-destructive lifestyle	Functional (veins, bones)
↑Irreversible↑	Unawareness	Organized (sclerosis, porosis)
--------------------------	Medicating disease	Curable
↓Reversible↓	↓	↑Reversible↑
Environmental stresses	Maturity	--------------------------
Lifestyle	Aging	↓Irreversible↓
Behavior	Rehabilitation	Debilitating
Sense of meaning in life	Living with disease	Incurable/Fatal
	Death	Death

A human life starts from birth and ends in death. Terminal disease is the pathological condition just before death. This fatal disease results from organized disease. Organized disease does not develop abruptly, but harbors previous conditions before it materializes pathologically. These can be called functional diseases, affected by aging, life-style, and "awareness" (alexithymia, alexisomia, and loss of life meaning).

(Nagata, K., V5, 1995)

treatment." This is the typical attitude of modern medicine towards "unorganized disease." However, when the functional disease finally manifests as an organized disease, it is often too late; Western medicine has little or no recourse. Similarly, modern medicine lacks adequate methods to cope with the side effects it causes. By contrast, traditional Oriental medicine can complement and overcome such shortcomings of current Western medicine.

Functional Disease: Unorganized Disease

The pioneer of medical interviews, Michael Balint (1957), propounded that "The most important role of a practitioner is to treat patients while their illness is still in an unorganized state." Balint meant that doctors should diagnose patients and initiate treatment during the pre-clinical (ill-health) stage. Current

Western medicine, based on anatomy and pathology, is very strong in diagnosis and treatment of organized diseases, but lacks satisfying diagnostic methods or treatments for functional diseases in the pre-clinical stage.

For over 3,000 years, traditional Oriental medicine has held that the best doctors cure unorganized conditions, and has regarded preventive medicine as its most important objective. Traditional Oriental medicine has provided treatments to ensure long and healthy life. Providing treatment at the stage of unorganized diseases is also essential to improve the QOL of patients with fatal diseases including cancer, myocardial infarction, and cerebral infarction.

One primary diagnostic technique of traditional Oriental medicine is empirical observation of vital fluid flow. The Japanese term *ketsu* itself refers to the whole dynamic homeostatic mechanism protecting the living body, including blood, hemodynamics (blood circulation), and autonomic nervous, immunological, and endocrinological systems. The term *Oketsu* literally means "stagnant blood"—a condition characterized by disturbed circulation of *ketsu*, the red fluids circulating in the living body. Traditional Oriental medicine actively investigates such disturbed hemodynamics.

Stagnation of blood flow may be local or generalized, but inevitably precedes more serious problems. For example, locally disturbed blood flow may induce gastric ulcers or stiff shoulders. In the living body, the local condition is always connected to systemic conditions. This is very different from inanimate systems; for example in the case of a car trouble, mere replacement of worn parts may be thought to solve a problem. By contrast, the oriental approach sees feathered tires and burned brake pads as symptomatic of a style of reckless driving that might advise reeducation of the living human driver lest sudden starts, stops, and turns lead to worse mishaps.

When blood flow is widely disturbed, it may presage a variety of potentially fatal diseases. Even diseases such as cancer, cerebral infarction and myocardial infarction represent the ultimate results of disturbed blood flow. Disturbed blood flow is not the sole or direct cause of fatal diseases, but it can serve as a diagnostic warning sign thereof. Before any disease progresses into its visible stages, a variety of symptoms can be seen; patients complain of symptoms such as loss of appetite, constipation, headache, stomach ache, dizziness or vertigo, insomnia, fatigue, difficulty in getting up in the morning. Neither doctors nor patients readily know which medical specialist to consult for such apparently general and common complaints, but such patients are rapidly increasing in number. To evaluate such patients comprehensively, we have introduced the concept of *Oketsu* diagnosis based on observable physical symptoms and urinalysis. We have developed a questionnaire form that facilitates our diagnosis (Nagata, 1995). Table 3 shows the criteria diagnostic of *Oketsu* syndrome.

Scientific Evaluation of *Oketsu*

In Oriental medicine, *Oketsu* is a complex symptomatology, so it is difficult to explain its pathophysiology in a few words. However, it mainly indicates poor hemodynamic condition.

For example, hemodynamic parameters determined in *Oketsu* patients revealed that heart rate (cardiac output in standing position) was significantly decreased; total peripheral resistance was elevated in patients with serious *Oketsu*. Patients with *Oketsu* also exhibit significantly increased platelet functions (releasing reaction: ß-TG, PF4). It is often observed that blood viscosity increases in *Oketsu* condition. Compared to healthy control groups, patients with *Oketsu* show seriously reduced serum levels of coenzyme Q10 (that produces adenosine triphosphate and controls free radicals); these findings correlate with their reductions in heart rate. Administering coenzyme Q10 to patients with *Oketsu* normalizes both their coenzyme Q10 serum levels and their *Oketsu*. Chinese herbal formulas such as *Toukaku-joukitou*, *Keishibuku-ryogan*, and *Toukishaku-yakusan* also serve to normalize the poor hemodynamics associated with *Oketsu* condition.

Comprehensive Medicine

Table 3: Diagnostic criteria of Oketsu Syndrome

Symptoms	Male	Female
Dark rings around the eyes	10	10
Discoloration (darkening) of the face	2	2
Rough skin	2	5
Dark red discoloration of lips	2	2
Dark red discoloration of gums	10	5
Purple discoloration of the tongue	10	10
Telangiectasis, vascular spiders	5	5
Susceptibility to subcutaneous bleeding	2	10
Redness of palms, palm erythema	2	5
Tenderness of the left navel region	5	5
Tenderness of the right navel region	10	10
Tenderness under the navel region	5	5
Tenderness of the iliocecal region	5	2
Tenderness of the sigmoid colon region	5	5
Tenderness of the hypochondrial region	5	5
Hemorrhoids	10	5
Dysmenorrhea		10

> 20 points or less: Non-*Oketsu* Related Condition
> 21 points and above: *Oketsu* Condition
> 40 points and above: Severe *Oketsu* Condition

(Terasawa, et. al.)

Oketsu and Unorganized Disease

In view of these findings, *Oketsu* condition may be said to represent prepathological but decreased cardiac function, or pathologically unorganized preconditions of myocardial or cerebral infarction. For example, serious *Oketsu* condition presages many cases of sudden death syndrome. In most of these cases, patients are not aware of their condition and leave it untreated. Such patients often are so busily devoted to their work that they do not pay attention to their deteriorating physical condition. Here we find psychosomatic problems such as hyper-adaptation, loss of somatic sensation, loss of emotion, and loss of meaning.

People totally devoted to achieve success in their business become hyper-adapted to urban industrial society and lifestyle, and so may lose touch with changes in their own emotions and physical conditions. These conditions are called alexithymia (loss of emotion) and alexisomia (loss of somatic sensation). It is possible to alert patients to their alexisomia through the traditional oriental medical concept of *Oketsu* diagnosis. Here is one place where traditional oriental medicine and modern psychosomatic medicine can cooperate to save patients from such conditions.

Sensitivity to one's physical condition can be cultivated, for example, by carefully observing one's appearance in the mirror while shaving or applying makeup in the morning. We doctors should educate patients about *Oketsu* to encourage their self-monitoring. In addition, for early detection and diagnosis of functional diseases, we should utilize *Oketsu* just like other vital signs in our daily practice of medicine. Detection of functional disease is but one way of recognizing unorganized disease. Not only *Oketsu* but also many other traditional Oriental medicinal concepts such as *Suitai* (or *Suidoku*: intracellular fluid retention) enable people to become aware of changes in their physical and mental condition. Here is the way to recover healthy condition from a condition of functional disease. This is the wisdom of the Orient. But now let us turn to some clinical cases that exemplify the theory we have been discussing.

Clinical Case 1: Sudden Death of a Businessman Over-Adapted to Stresses

The patient was a 45-year-old businessman of a trading company. Although his periodical medical checkups had diagnosed him as having mild hypertension, slight diabetes mellitus, and fatty liver, he was not thought to require any treatment.

His past history was unremarkable. His family medical history showed that his father had died from cerebral infarction at the age of 42, and his mother from pulmonary tuberculosis. The patient himself had wanted to become a certified public accountant. However, as his father died while he was a high school student, he had to quit high school to take a job to earn the money to provide education for his younger brothers. While continuing this job, he earned both his high school diploma and even a college degree by going to night school. But his wife later reported that he used to mutter to himself that he wished he had become a certified public accountant.

He became a capable, competent, diligent businessman, seldom absent from work. He earned a high reputation and was repeatedly commended by his company. He was known as a hard-working but sociable boss. He never turned down a work assignment. He made many business trips for his company, traveling almost every week, and flying overseas every month. He experienced many transfers within his company and worked continuously for 20 years at a local branch, living apart from his wife and family. He worked feverishly and earned a high salary, but did not enjoy his work, always feeling pressured by work and stressed by human relations. To relieve himself from these problems and stresses, he indulged in drinking, smoking, and sometimes gambling all night. As he lived alone in the town near his branch office, he was not regular in his lifestyle. Forgoing sleep and rest, he worked day and night for two years to complete an important project for his company. His devotion brought the project to a smashing success, but in the party thrown to celebrate that success, he collapsed and died suddenly of a heart attack.

His wife and family lived near my university hospital; she had hypertension, for which we treated her. One day when he happened to be home visiting his family, his wife noticed that his face color was very bad. As he himself complained of persistent headache, stiff shoulders, nausea and dizziness, his wife visited me at our hospital with her husband. Our general examination and medical laboratory tests revealed no pathological problems at all except incipient diabetes mellitus and fatty liver.

Then we conducted "Schellong's tilting test" in order to examine hemodynamic changes in the response of his autonomic nervous system. His supine blood pressure was 138/85 mmHg, which was normal, but blood pressure after 10 minutes of tilting was 195/139 mmHg, elevating gradually, indicating orthostatic hypertension. [The hemodynamic reason of elevating blood pressure was the increase of stroke volume after tilting, which means the stimulation of the inotropic action of the cardiac sympathetic nerve.] This orthostatic hypertension appears frequently in patients with lacunae cerebral infarctions. This type of cerebral infarction can seldom be detected by cerebral CT (computed tomography), but only by MRI (magnetic resonance imaging). In fact, MRI findings revealed that indeed he had multiple lacunae cerebral infarctions as our *Oketsu* diagnosis predicted.

When we examine for orthostatic regulation, in addition to measuring blood pressure, we also routinely perform Korotkoff's soundgram (KSG). Korotkoff's sound is readily audible when blood pressure is measured with a stethoscope; KSG is Korotkoff's sound mechanically graphed and analyzed into hemodynamic data. We found this patient's KSG was normal in supine position, but showed a specific "Right-Angled Triangle Type" immediately after he stood up, indicating that the blood flow to his cerebral and/or coronary artery decreased briefly but notably with the strain of tilting. The KSG reveals this functional reaction that appears only transitorily when the tilting test stimulates the autonomic nervous system. Although his EKG showed no abnormality, he displayed severe *Oketsu* syndrome as diagnosed by the methods of traditional Oriental medicine. His poor complexion that alarmed his wife was one symptom of his *Oketsu* syndrome.

He was too busy with his work every day, and he over-adapted because of his pursuit of success. To escape from his accumulated stresses, he spent a self-destructive life. Psychosomatically he had clearly lost his own affection, somatic sensation, and sense of meaning in life. This alexithymic and alexisomic condition resulted from his over-adaptation to his circumstances. Even under such circumstances, there is a possibility the patient may recuperate if he pursues a clear purpose or finds meaning in his life. Unluckily for this man, the work he was doing was not very meaningful for him. Due to his type A behavior and personality, he was at a high risk for coronary disease. Moreover he was in a slightly depressive condition.

We explained that he needed rest and should be hospitalized to receive treatment. We further told him that there was a danger that he would face irreversible cerebral infarction if he failed to change his lifestyle. He listened to our explanation half in doubt. As he was hardly persuaded, I prescribed him some drugs, including a ß-blocker and antidepressant, and wrote a referral letter to a physician near his business site. I urged him to receive treatment immediately as an inpatient. In spite of this, he neglected our warning and continued his work and self-destructive lifestyle.

The consequence was his death from heart attack. Only his wife's regret remained. Japanese doctors frequently see such patients these days; such sudden deaths from overwork *(Karoushi)* have come to constitute a social problem in Japan.

Four Defects of Western Cathartic Medicine

Modern Western medicine faces four weak areas compared to complementary medicine. Put simply, they are (1) public distrust of the medical profession; (2) inability to diagnose and treat functional disabilities and diseases in their early stages; (3) side effects of medical treatment of organized diseases; and (4) inappropriate care for terminal and very elderly patients. In the confused medical world today, improvement of terminal care is also an important task whose necessity has long been advocated, but propagation is regrettably slow. In such cases, complementary approaches

(Japanese: *Hohou*) are helpful to improve patients' QOL. Current Western medicine has few complementary approaches compared to traditional Oriental and psychosomatic medicine. To obtain homeostatic efficacy, it is essential to maintain a good balance between complementary approaches and cathartic approaches.

The Role of Logotherapy (Existential Analysis) in Comprehensive Medicine

One psychosomatic approach that we recommend is Victor Frankl's "logotherapy" (an existential psychological analysis helping the patient find meaning in life (Frankl, 1959). To face death and the dying process without losing dignity, we must begin with a subjective awareness of the meanings of one's life. The "life review interview" is one such method. We sometimes encounter patients who have overcome terminal cancer and created new lives for themselves by logotherapeutic approaches. One of the features commonly seen in such patients is that they achieved a shift from negative stubbornness to a positively flexible attitude toward life.

Such a lifestyle change cannot be achieved by chance (it is not a miracle), nor does it result from psychotherapy alone. Quality care guaranteeing good appetite, sound sleep, and pain control is prerequisite. Such comprehensive care can be achieved only when both the patient's family and the hospital coordinate their efforts toward the same improvement of QOL. Besides these comprehensive approaches from the family and the hospital, individual patients must gain an understanding of their important or peak experiences, and awareness of their interconnectedness with significant others. Through such efforts, we have sometimes attained really high levels of QOL even for patients diagnosed as terminal.

To this end, caregivers should "Never, never, never give up," (Churchill), should "nurture every chance of growth until the last moment of life" (Kübler-Ross), and should provide hope to patients while respecting their autonomy.

Both the prospect of death and the dying process are great stresses to humans. Approaches to cope with such stresses include "fighting," "escaping," and "living with disease." The most humanistic approach to coping is "to learn to live with disease" (to conquer disease by agreeing to live with it).

Complementarity of Western, Traditional Oriental, and Psychosomatic Medicine

All current Western medicine, traditional Oriental medicine, and psychosomatic medicine aim at the same goal; however, they differ in indication, based on their differences in fundamental viewpoint, philosophy, methodology and history.

Based on the enlightenment ideals of analysis, reproducibility, and universality, modern biochemical medicine uses physical and chemical examinations and diagnostic imaging techniques like X-rays, CT scans, MRI, and ultrasound. This scientific worldview has led to the development of surgical methods based on techniques such as anesthesia and tumor resection, and antibiotic therapy for bacterial infections. In oriental terms, this medicine is advanced in cathartic approaches including removal, resection, tapping, crushing, and is mainly indicated for organized diseases, where it produces clear-cut therapeutic results. However, Western medicine often produces pronounced side effects.

Traditional Oriental medicine tries to understand patients comprehensively and conceptually, beginning with four kinds of close observation of patients: watching, smelling, listening, and touching. It always views patients holistically, and its main indications are functional diseases and terminal diseases. Traditional Oriental medicine characteristically maintains a good balance between cathartic approaches and complementary approaches. Oriental medicine appears inferior to Western medicine in that its therapeutic effects are not immediately evident, and it may be less effective for already organized and acute diseases.

At once analytical and extensive, psychosomatic medicine also grasps patients from a comprehensive viewpoint that aims to balance somatic and psycho-social-existential approaches. Psychosomatic medicine becomes even more effective when it incorporates care (medical support) in addition to cure (medical healing). Psychosomatic medicine has both Western and Oriental characteristics, cultivating patients' awareness and behavioral modification of distorted, self-destructive lifestyles. For example, relaxation by autogenic training is useful to relieve a patient from functional diseases. Although psychosomatic medicine is not so effective in the treatment of acute or organized diseases, the medical profession needs to pay attention to patients' psychological, social, and existential problems that affect their immunity and recovery.

Figure 2 shows the efficacy curves of 3 medical approaches. Ideally, doctors would mutually respect and appropriately utilize these three medical approaches, understanding the indications and limitations of the respective systems.

Clinical Case 2: A Stout-Hearted Old Woman Who Overcame Cancer

The patient was an eighty-three year old woman, afflicted with severe neck and shoulder pain and severe coughs in winter. She was diagnosed to have adenoid cystic carcinoma of the salivary gland and its pulmonary metastases. She had a tumorous mass of 4 cm in diameter in the right submaxilla, involving the submaxillary bone and infiltrated to the blood vessels of the neck area. Of course these lesions caused her much pain. Her lungs displayed innumerable metastatic lesions, the source of her incessant coughing. With a sigh, a university hospital specialist informed her family that it was too late; that she could not survive even three months.

The patient was renowned for being an obstinate old woman. When she was still young, her husband had died in World War II, so she raised her three daughters by herself. Unfortunately, her second daughter was both mentally and physically disabled. The patient struggled desperately, because she had promised her husband on his deathbed that she would raise this second daughter to the last. So she protected this pitiful but beloved child by herself, not entrusting her care to anyone. Therefore, she had never allowed herself to travel, never boarded a plane or long-distance train. She never let her other daughters take care of this disabled

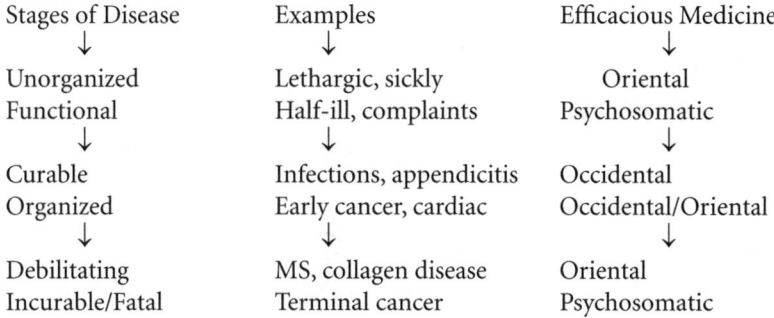

Figure 2. Therapeutic Efficacy of Occidental, Oriental, and Psychosomatic Medicine

Stages of Disease ↓	Examples ↓	Efficacious Medicine ↓
Unorganized Functional ↓	Lethargic, sickly Half-ill, complaints ↓	Oriental Psychosomatic ↓
Curable Organized ↓	Infections, appendicitis Early cancer, cardiac ↓	Occidental Occidental/Oriental ↓
Debilitating Incurable/Fatal	MS, collagen disease Terminal cancer	Oriental Psychosomatic

daughter, even though they volunteered eagerly.

She often told herself, "I could never apologize to my departed husband if I were to ask others to take care of my second daughter. I will take care of her to the last."

For this reason, she lamented that she got ill. The more she regretted her illness, the more her pain intensified. At the outpatient service, she begged me, "Doctor, I can't stand the pain. Please do something to help me. I must not die now!"

Fortunately, the excruciating pain in her submaxilla was almost completely alleviated by my pain point block, a nerve block producing immediate effects by injecting local anesthetic every centimeter around the tumor.

At about that time, her younger brother died in Hokkaido,

1,000 km north of Tokyo. After anguished consideration, for the first time in her life, she asked her first daughter's family to take care of her disabled second daughter, so that she could fly to Hokkaido to attend her brother's funeral. Of course the funeral was a sad event, but she was deeply impressed by the journey. The beautiful natural scenery of Hokkaido in the misty early spring as seen from the airplane really fascinated her, and she resolved to bring her second daughter to see that wonderful scenery. It was a supreme and sublime experience. When she came back from Hokkaido full of apprehensions about her second daughter, she was surprised to see how well her second daughter got along with the family of her first daughter.

She reflected to herself; she realized that she had protected her daughter too much. As a result, she had narrowed the world in which her second daughter lived, and she had made her own life monotonously flat.

She changed herself when she was already eighty-three years old. She reformed her sedentary and obstinate character and became active and gentle. She awoke to the meaning as well as the responsibility of her life, and chose to enjoy her own life with her disabled daughter. She yearned to recover her good health as soon as possible, to relish her life again for her own sake as well as for her second daughter.

One day she came to us and requested hospitalization. I prescribed analgesic therapy by pain point block, Oriental herbal formulae (*Juzentaihotou* with red ginseng)) with coenzyme Q10, and logotherapy (psychotherapy to make the patient aware of meaning of her own life and to find value in the experiences the patient had lived through). We conducted daily life review interviews (following Balint and Frankl) to reconceptualize her life experiences and help her find the meaning in her remaining life.

Then her submaxillary cancer miraculously went into remission, and the progression of her lung metastases stopped. Her pain and coughs disappeared as if she had never had such an attack.

When she was discharged from our hospital 2 months later, surprisingly she had gained 4 kg of body weight! More than anything, she became a cheerful old woman who laughed often. She survived nine and a half years after she had been sentenced to a three-month lifetime. She was not bedridden but spent happy days full of laughter and a valuable life worth living with her family. Of course, she visited Hokkaido again with her disabled second daughter.

QOL of Terminally Ill Cancer Patients with Intractable Pain

In Japan, we examined the QOL status of 21 cases of terminally ill cancer patients with incurable pain by our "QOL Questionnaire." Their QOL was miserable. These patients had already completed cathartic approaches such as operations, radiation, and chemotherapy, but their conditions had declined with severe pain. After thoroughgoing informed consent, we introduced a wide array of complementary methods to alleviate their intractable pain, specifically: morphine, coenzyme Q10, Oriental herbal formula (*Juzentaihotou* with red ginseng, a standard herbal formula for weakened patients), and logotherapy. Four weeks after beginning our complementary care, their pain and appetite had improved statistically. Eight weeks later, other items of QOL improved, and no worsened items were found!

I called the old lady's case "miraculous," but in fact it is merely the natural outcome of performing proper comprehensive medical care.

Natural Remission of Cancer

More than 20 years ago, Yujiro Ikemi described the natural remission of cancer in his paper entitled "Psychosomatic consideration of cancer patients who have made a narrow escape from death" (Ikemi, 1975). Just before his own passing, Dr. Ikemi was invited to give a special lecture at the "First International Conference on

Natural Remission of Cancer" at the University of Heidelberg in April of 1997. According to Ikemi's paper, among patients with natural reduction in cancer tumor size, one fourth became devoted to their life work, and another quarter came to have religious consciousness. These cases also evidenced remarkable immunological and antiallergenic effects (Table 4).

Table 4: Psychological and somatic conditions in patients with spontaneous regression of cancer

Physiological effects	Psycho-social shift				Total
	Religious Awareness	Existential shift	Support from family	Devotion to lifework	
Endocrinological effects	2		2	1	5
Immunological or allergic reactions	3	4	2	3	12
Incomplete resection of cancerous tissue	2		1	2	5
Decreased nutrition to cancerous tissue		1			1
Infection and fever		1			1
Total	7	6	5	6	24

(by Ikemi, Y.)

Conditions for Existential Shift

The term "existential shift" was first used in connection with cancer remission by the American psychologist George Booth (1973). In fact, some patients with intractable cancer or neurological diseases have successfully achieved such existential shifts. Such existential shifts cannot be obtained in animal experiments, but are possible only for humans. What conditions lead patients to such existential shifts? Our medical team has researched these phenomena.

Among patients in our daily practice who reached the status of "living with disease," we found the following common features:

1) After they became ill, they experience some "peak experience"—being deeply impressed by beautiful nature or art, gaining a bodily sense of the joy of living, realizing their lives are deeply interconnected with the support of many persons.
2) Such bodily sense leads patients to recognize that each person is "being kept alive" and has "living life." Thus patients become aware of their meanings within personal relationships and histories. Instead of merely bemoaning their illnesses, they come to consider how to live despite their diseases.
3) Such recognition leads patients to feel gratitude and joy in encounters with others, because they interpret each encounter as a unique opportunity in their life. Then patients face their lives less pessimistically, but rather actively—to live their lives as fully as they can—and with humor, coming to laugh readily at the slightest occasion.
4) Families', doctors', and nurses' cooperation to provide humanistic, comprehensive medicine minimizes patients' distrust of medicine, and doctors establish good relations with their patients.
5) The doctor is familiar with comprehensive medicine and provides medical treatment that relieves pain and increases patients' appetites.
6) The doctors integrate their practice of modern medical methods with complementary treatments (including Chinese herbal supplements, acupuncture, logotherapeutic psychological treatment, and hot spa treatment) in a justifiable manner, and the patients accept them (see Table 1).
7) As a result of such treatment, patients rediscover the meaning of their lives, becoming aware of their responsibility in living and of their freedom to change their behavior patterns. Through such processes, patients change their attitudes from stubbornness to gentle persistence.

Scientific Evaluation of "Living With Disease"

Humans always face stressors, which stimulate the adrenocortical area of our pituitary glands to release ACTH (adrenocorticotropic hormones), producing cortisol. (We can measure cortisol levels by measuring its metabolite 17-OHCS (hereafter "OH") found in urine after metabolism.) Cortisol in turn draws on other bodily tissues to produce glucose to generate energy to resist stress. As a result, cortisol causes wear and tear to the living body; excessive cortisol production leads to various diseases such as diabetes and arteriosclerosis. Repetition of such wear and tear eventually results in death, so living bodies protect and restore themselves against this. However, the substances and mechanisms of stress protection have remained a mystery for a long time. Recently scientists have shown that DHEA-S (dehydroepiandrosterone sulfate) is the hormone of "restoration" which resists the "deterioration" caused by cortisol.

DHEA-S is a precursor of adrenogenic hormones. It builds immunity, exerts anabolic effects, biosynthesizes proteins in the body, controls arteriosclerosis, increases physical strength and vitality, elevates mood, and promotes restful sleep. In addition, DHEA-S maintains the functions of neurocytes and increases the susceptibility of peripheral cells to insulin. All of these reactions are beneficial to bodily functions (Nishikaze, 1993). DHEA-S is biosynthesized in the adrenals and testicles as well as in the brain and skin, but the brain produces more DHEA-S than other organs. When a living body is exhausted by stress, the most important mechanism to restore an exhausted body is production of DHEA-S. The levels of a person's DHEA-S can easily be measured by measuring its urinary metabolites 17-KS-S (hereafter "S"), originally discovered by H. Nishikaze and E. Furuya (1978; confirmed in 1985 version). The level of "S" decreases with aging or illness. In a person's early twenties, the level of "S" reaches its peak, decreasing thereafter with age. Diseases such as hypotension, hypertension, diabetes, cancer, and myocardial infarction radically reduce the level of "S."

There are a variety of methods available for examination prior to prescribing drugs or cathartic operations. Conventional laboratory tests are disease-specific; for example, if liver tests reveal elevations in GOT and GPT, liver dysfunction is suspected. However, there were few scientific methods available for evaluations in complementary medicine. For many years, doctors have sought an objective method of verifying the ratio of stress to the body's resistance to stress. Recently, we have discovered an extremely simple and accurate means of doing so, using the urinary metabolites of DHEA-S and cortisol, "S" and "OH" respectively. The DHEA-S metabolite "S" reflects the patient's level of stress-resistance and vitality, while the cortisol metabolite "OH" reflects the patient's exposure to stress. Thus the "S"/"OH" ratio indicates the patient's "relative stress condition." By introduction of the "S"/"OH" ratio, we can determine when it is beneficial to apply complementary approaches. This is not a disease-specific diagnostic measure, but rather objectively shows the patient's stress-resistance and health level.

Thus "S," "OH" and "S"/"OH" are important parameters for evaluation of complementary approach. A doctor's decision of whether to choose a complementary approach or a cathartic approach after assessment of patient's condition has generally depended on the doctor's experience and instincts. There was no objective method for this kind of assessment. This was one main cause for the delay in propagation of Oriental medicine. However, our introduction of "S," "OH" and "S"/"OH" has made objective assessment possible.

We followed up the "S"/"OH" ratio of 11 patients with terminal cancer who reached the state of "living with their disease" using complementary drugs and logotherapeutic approaches, for about one year. The results we obtained were just as previously hypothesized: their initially low urinary levels of 17-KS-S gradually increased, and one year later their improved QOL was reflected by increases in urinary levels of their 17-KS-S. However, those patients with cancer who had strong anxiety also showed persistently elevated 17-OHCS levels.

Figure 3: Changes in "S," "OH," and "S"/"OH" by Supplementary Treatments

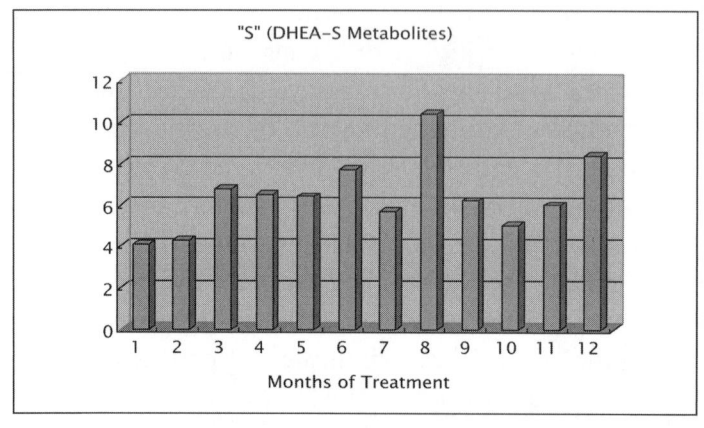

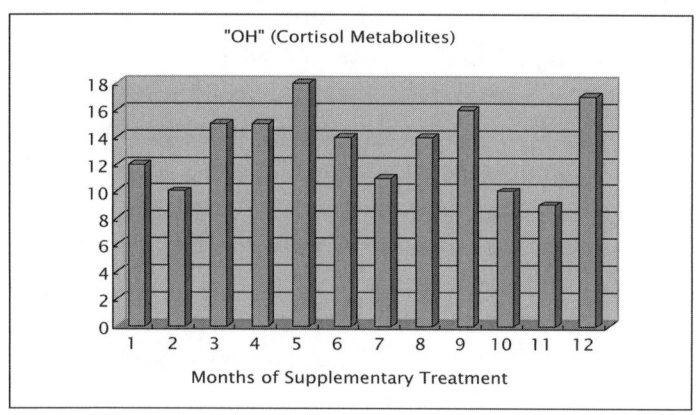

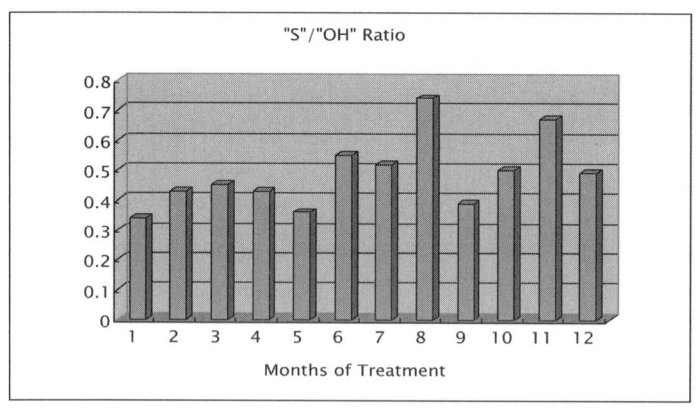

As can be clearly seen from the general adaptation syndrome described by Selye, (1974), even a single disease changes over time in the life of a patient. The period of youth, abounding in physical strength, is a stage of high resistance. But after this period, one slowly moves into phases of decreased physical strength. Naturally, we doctors must differentiate our treatment approaches to individual patients' circumstances. Sometimes we hear that anticancer drugs were administered to a patient with terminal cancer until the very morning of the day of death. This is the shortcoming of providing treatment based only on laboratory diagnoses, without grasping the patient's levels of strength or stress resistance.

Yujiro Ikemi advocated individualized treatment, meaning that doctors should first grasp the bio-psycho-socio-existential circumstances unique to the patient, and secondly determine the specific method of treatment considering the patient's stage and strength. If a doctor establishes an erroneous diagnosis at this period, the treatment may overtax the physical strength of the patient, breaking the balance. Then, the meaning of treatment decreases and the patient will be troubled or even killed by the side effects. Therefore, to provide individualized and safe treatment, correct diagnosis not only of the disease itself, but also of the patient's bodily strength and stress resistance is indispensable to grasp patients' conditions. Here, "S," "OH" and "S"/"OH" ratios can serve as invaluable objective aids in medical decision-making. The "S," "OH" and "S"/OH" ratios are important not only for initial assessment of patients, but also for follow-up evaluation of the effects of the treatments we doctors prescribe.

Wisdom to Overcome Shortcomings of Current Western Medicine: Complementary Approaches

Here I should like to reconsider some shortcomings of current Western medicine described above. We have identified four points that current Western medicine should overcome:

1) Public distrust of the medical profession
2) Inability to diagnose and treat functional disabilities and diseases in their early stages
3) Side effects of medical treatment of organized diseases
4) Inappropriate care for terminal and very elderly patients.

Solutions of problems (2) through (4) will largely resolve the distrust in (1). Then what points are common to items (2) and (3)? Fatigue is a typical indicator of the change from a healthy condition to a condition of functional disease (half-healthy/half-ill). Fatigue indicates reduction in physical strength and homeostasis in general.

If a patient suffers from side effects while receiving medical treatment, this suggests that the cathartic treatment (such as chemotherapy, surgery, radiotherapy, etc.) outstrips the patient's bodily homeostasis mechanisms. So medical treatment that is helpful for a certain part of the body produces adverse side-effects in other parts of the body. Extreme reduction in physical strength and homeostasis appear can ultimately lead to fatal pathological conditions (too late to be cured) at the terminal stage.

The common characteristic of these three points is that patients have reduced physical strength or spirit; it is the job of complementary approaches to improve the QOL of these patients. Regrettably, current Western medicine does not use many complementary approaches. By contrast, traditional Oriental medicine and psychosomatic medicine have a number of complementary approaches, as shown in Table 1. Among complementary approaches, there are somatic approaches and psychological approaches, besides adjustments of lifestyle such as dietary habits, exercise, and sleep. Such complementary approaches are invaluable to increase patients' DHEA-S levels. In the United States, an increasing number of people take DHEA-S supplements, since their beneficial effect was reported in an October 1996 issue of *Newsweek*. Little is known about the side effects of orally administered DHEA-S supplements. However, you do not have to purchase the drug to increase DHEA-S, as there are many healthier methods available. (Various methods to increase DHEA-S are shown in Table 5.) Creation of a healthy lifestyle invariably results in elevations of DHEA-S levels.

Table 5: Methods to increase DHEA-S (by complementary approaches)

1. Regular lifestyle and healthy habits
    a) Meals (especially breakfasts)
    b) Exercise (at least 3 times a week)
    c) Sound sleep
2. Physical supplements
    a) Complementary agents (Oriental herbs, *Juzentaihotou*, red ginseng, vitamins, co-Q10)
    b) Hot spa baths, natural rest and recovery
    c) Complementary acupuncture, massage
    d) Comfortable treatment, use of complementary medical devices
    e) DHEA(-S) itself
3. Psychological supplements
    a) Having awareness of meaning of life (taking responsibility for free choice)
    b) Peak experiences
    c) Recognition of value of own life supported by surroundings
    d) Joy of "for this time only"
    e) Consider "how" rather than "why"

Need → **Sufficient care**
　　　→ **Balance between complementary and cathartic approaches**

Doctors too should familiarize themselves with complementary approaches to increase homeostasis. We can overcome some shortcomings of current Western medicine by introducing complementary approaches. For example, we have often forestalled or offset the side effects of anti-tumor drugs by using complementary drugs such as *Juzentaihotou,* red ginseng, and coenzyme Q10 in anti-cancer therapy. Another complementary herbal formulae called Saireito is similarly effective to prevent side effects of steroid hormones. These methods have repeatedly been shown effective in improving QOL and increasing the 17-KS-S levels described above.

This is not a problem of choosing between Western and Oriental approaches. Doctors as well as patients must strive for a good balance of cathartic and complementary approaches to achieve homeostasis, or overall bodily benefit. Introduction of the concepts of traditional Oriental medicine is invaluable to make current Western medicine even more effective and more complete.

Conclusion

The most important complementary component in treating exhausted and debilitated patients is doctors' attitude. The effects of a doctor's loving concern on a debilitated patient cannot be overestimated (Balint, 1957). The doctor's sympathy and care for exhausted patients is the very "therapeutic self" advocated by Watkins (1978).

Entering the 21st century, it is essential that we incorporate traditional Oriental medicine and psychosomatic medicine into current Western medicine, with mutual respect. Such incorporation of medical practice and theory can best be accomplished in the context of comprehensive medicine (Nagata, 2000). This is our responsibility as medical professionals, and a growing community of informed patients is coming to expect as much.

References

Balint, M. (1957). *The Doctor, His Patient, and the Illness.* London: M. J. Pittman.

Booth, G. (1973). "Psychological aspects of 'spontaneous' regression of cancer." *American Journal of Psychoanalysis,* 1, 303–317.

Day, S.B., Lolas, F., & Kusinitz, M. (eds.). (1980). *Biopsychosocial Health.* New York: The International Foundation for Biosocial Development and Human Health, p. 181f.

Frankl, V. E. (1959). *Man's Search for Meaning: an Introduction to Logotherapy.* Boston: Beacon Press, p. 237f.

Furuya, E., Graef, V., & Nishikaze, O. (1978). "An improved method based on the Porter-Silber reaction for determining 17-hydroxycorticosteroids in urine." *Analytical Biochemistry,* 90, 644–65.

Ikemi, Y., Nakagawa, T., & Sugita, M. (1975). "Psychosomatic consideration of cancer patients who have made a narrow escape from death." *Dynamic Psychiatry,* 31, 77–9.

Nagata, K. (1992). "Quality of life variables as new health indicators." In S. Araki, ed., *Behavioral Medicine: An Integrated Biobehavioral Approach to Health and Illness.* Amsterdam: Elsevier, 309–319.

Nagata, K. (1995). "Comprehensive medicine based on bio-psycho-socio-existential medicine." *Comprehensive Medicine* (Japan), 1(1), 15–32.

Nagata, K. (1996). "Psychosomatic medicine: An integrator of Western and Oriental medicine in the context of comprehensive medicine." In Y. Ikemi. ed., *Integration of Eastern and Western Psychosomatic Medicine.* Fukuoka: Kyushu University Press, 189–214.

Nagata, K. (2000). *Comprehensive Medicine: Bio-psycho-social Medicine, An Oriental & Western Overview.* New York: International Foundation for Biosocial Development and Human Health.

Nishikaze, O., & Iwata, J. (1985). "A direct determination of sulfate conjugates of 17-oxosteroids in urine by use of benzyltributylammonium chloride—without solvolysis and enzymatic hydrolysis." *Japan Journal of Clinical Chemistry,* 14, 204–207.

Nishikaze, O. (1993) "The XIIth UOEA symposium on 'Stress Proteins,'whole body responses to stress: adrenocortical adaptation to stress in humans", *JUOEH,* 15: 264–268.

Selye, H. (1974). *Stress without Distress.* New York: Lippincott.

Watkins, J. G. (1978). *The Therapeutic Self Developing Resonance.* New York: Human Sciences Press.

11.

The Changing Faces of Disease and Psycho-Spiritual Healing

Carl Becker, Ph.D., D.Litt.
Integrated Human Sciences, Kyoto University, Japan

Introduction

No one wants to fall critically ill. Yet no one can predict a life-threatening illness. Before World War II, bacteria carried by insects, vermin, or dirty water caused most fatal illnesses. To prevent fatal diseases, it was only necessary to eliminate their carriers and boil the water. People who had contracted diseases would either recover or die in a few weeks. Today, most fatal diseases in advanced countries are not bacterial but diseases of lifestyle. They come neither from mosquito bites nor from dirty food, but from many years of stress, of breathing smoke, drinking chemicals, eating food coloring, preservatives, too much sugar, fat, and salt. Just as they are not caused quickly, such diseases cannot be cured quickly. They often involve years of slow degeneration of body and brain. This poses dilemmas both for society and for doctors.

Ironically, Asian as well as western doctors still tend to use the same remedies which worked against infectious diseases: rest, nutrition, drugs, and quarantine. However effective these approaches may be against hostile bacteria, they have little effect on diseases like cancer and arteriosclerosis that are caused not by invasive bugs, but by decades of diet, lifestyle, and character traits. A few weeks of drugs and rest cannot resuscitate elderly people from the effects of these new killers. All too often, such elderly patients are placed in care, not for weeks, but for years, while nurses try to rehabilitate them.

Society's dilemma arises from the tremendous costs of money, facilities, and manpower required for long-term terminal care. Health insurance was designed to cover the costs of treating simple diseases, accidents, childbirth—short-term problems that people commonly face. Neither governments nor private insurance can provide total long-term care and high-tech medicine for everyone. It is unfair to tax people who take good care of their health, in order to pay for the medical expenses of those who smoke and drink and risk their health. New approaches must include private insurance fitted to the desires and lifestyles of the insured; and health education to reduce the risk of unexpected health problems in later life.

Recognizing the inadequacy of modern medicine to overcome today's killer diseases, recent years have witnessed a burgeoning interest in alternative, complementary, holistic and preventive medicine. The tremendous economic implications of this move have attracted the interests of insurance companies, pharmaceutical industries, state and local governments. In America and Europe, vitamin, mineral, and herbal dietary supplements have become billion dollar businesses—and so have psychiatry, counseling, massage and acupuncture.

Non-medical healing is predicted to account for nearly half of the new jobs in the next generation. Massage therapists in the United States have already quadrupled in the past 10 years; and more than 100,000 new jobs are expected in the field of religious counseling and therapy in America alone! [Occupational Outlook Handbook @ www.bls.govlocohome.htm] Newspapers and magazines are filled with stories of how alternative therapies saved lives, marriages, and careers. American insurance companies have found that they save money by reimbursing patients who seek religious therapy and counseling rather than by reimbursing bills for medicine and hospitals.

Studies in medical sociology and medical ethics have repeatedly demonstrated that it is more cost-effective to devote monies to improving the sanitation and health education of the lower classes than to genetic and medical research or advanced high-tech medical technologies. Preventive payment for basic mental and physical health for the lower classes raises the health of the upper class on the average even more than paying the same amounts directly for the upper class' high-end medical treatments without aiding the whole population!

American research has shown that grief work counseling can economically improve the health of the surviving bereaved. Grief work counseling gathers the family and loved ones at monthly intervals, beginning several months prior to the patient's death, and continuing for several months thereafter. The counselor provides a place and atmosphere where people can discuss their fears and concerns, feelings of guilt and loss, grief and hope. Comparing the health and mortality of bereaved families who have experienced grief work counseling with those who have not, a surprising difference emerges. While uncounseled bereaved tend to inordinate rates of disease, accident, suicide and death, the rate of the counseled bereaved is no greater than that of the average population. This is not only interesting from a psychological point of view; it is also highly significant for the future of national health as well as economy. To heal diseases, accidents, and suicide attempts after they have occurred requires tremendous time and expense. Well-scheduled hours of counseling can prevent such tragedies, protecting the health of the bereaved families, and saving funds for insurance companies and government ministries of health and welfare.

These rapidly evolving social and economic phenomena prompt a reconsideration of the nature and value of traditional views of health, wellness, and illness.

Traditional Implications of Disease

Throughout most of history, people have recognized diseases not merely as occasions of physical pain or inconvenience, but as indications of a need to rethink and reform their mental attitudes, spiritual problems, or social lifestyles. Sickness poses an invaluable opportunity to reevaluate one's thoughts and actions. Whether the result of stress, anxiety, overwork, cold, unbalanced diet, overindulgence, lack of exercise, or whatever, a period of enforced inactivity and recuperation becomes a time of self-reflection in which to rebalance lifestyles, values, and interpersonal relationships as well.

From the perspective of traditional religions, illness constructively educates us like a rite of passage to further spiritual growth; it is not simply a physical inconvenience, a hindrance to the work of accumulating and consuming material things, in which no meaning nor learning is to be found. Indeed, it is when we get sick that we most begin to question why we are here, what life and death are all about, and how our present lifestyles might be mistaken. If we correct our physical discomforts with pain-killers and laxatives, we may fail to learn the lessons that we are not eating, sleeping, or exercising properly—and even possibly the lessons that our lives need more spiritual foundations. What a *waste* it would be if illness were simply considered an annoyance, "lost time" to be overcome with a pill or an injection, if no personal or existential insights were gained about lifestyle in the process!

So it is with aging. The body ages and declines in an irreversible and ineluctable process that should be a cause for reflection on our mortality. The Buddha tells the parable of the old man fallen into Hell. Yama, King of Hell, asks the man if he never met three heavenly messengers. When the old man denies having met heavenly messengers, Yama asks more directly, "Have you never met elderly, sick, or dying people?" When the man acknowledges that he has often met elderly, sick, and dying people, Yama admonishes, "You have come to Hell because you ignored their warning of your own aging, sickness, and mortality." (1 *Anguttara Nikaya* 3-62).

Attempts to deny the aging process, through surgery or liposuction, breast implants or hair transplants, are not only pathetically vain but fundamentally deluded and self-deluding. Loss of mental or physical strength and resiliency with age is certainly saddening, but how utterly depressing it would be if we learned nothing from this process, if deluded elders were to crave continually for eternal youth!

Western science and medicine, paradigmatically analytic, tend to underestimate the variety of factors that give rise to diseases and immunity impairment. Conversely, Buddhist, Taoist, and Eastern philosophies tend to see causes, not as singular, unique, or operating *in vacua*, but rather as multifold, interlinked, and dependent on a wide range of causal conditions. (While science understands this theoretically, it tends to simplification for methodological purposes.) A reduced human hubris and a more holistic understanding of human health as well as environmental integrity is encouraged by a re-reading of Eastern medical models. If medicine is a war on aging and disease, it is doomed to failure, because aging and disease can never be overcome. [This is a fundamental insight of Buddhism.] Western-trained doctors typically provide no spiritual care for their patients because they have been taught to rescue the body but not to counsel the soul when the body is intractable. A more humble understanding of the limitations of medicine and technology might lead to a more humane treatment of patients.

Disease is not only an occasion for personal self-reflection; in many societies, it becomes an occasion for social integration or re-socialization. In this view, just as Western medicine focuses too narrowly on particular organs or microorganisms to treat the whole person, so Western medicine focuses too narrowly on particular patients to treat the whole problem, which inevitably reflects aspects of the social environment and interpersonal interactions. There is a fundamental difference between the individual patient seeking out a doctor and the community rallying to treat an ailing member.

In Balian, Siberian, American Indian, and other societies, the sickness of one member is recognized as a physical and spiritual danger to the whole community. So the whole community gathers in response to the call. Witch doctors, wise women, or shamans interrogate both the sick person and all those connected to her. Then they depersonalize, and the voice of a higher being, nature spirit, or ancestor speaks through them to prescribe the apologies, purification ceremonies, or cooperative social rites required to heal not only the individual but the entire community. Traditional healing is a holistic and all-embracing sort of practice, in which native healers see spirits, communicate with nature, sense the feelings of their fellows (not "patients"), and interact telepathically and intuitively as a matter of course. (Edge, Eliade, Walsh.)

Some Westerners criticize the worldviews of original peoples as second-rate, "primitive" attempts at what Western doctors do professionally. In fact, we should recognize that many Western doctors achieve only second-rate, primitive attempts at the integrative psychosocial healing that shamans accomplish. Shamans are not conducting anything like Western medicine, nor are there "doctors and clients" in most societies. The people who come to shamans are not simply asking for cure of physical conditions; they are asking the shaman to help them "find their lives" (Krippner, 49), so that they may live more meaningfully, lovingly, joyously. It is this dimension of healing that is tragically missing from most Western medical practice.

Stan Krippner calls spiritual healing

> …beneficial to humanity rather than to one person, oriented toward service rather than toward fame and fortune, supportive of love and empowerment rather than fostering fear and negativity, allowing for choice rather than demanding obedience, cognizant of a higher power rather than claiming ultimate authority for itself, presenting knowledge creatively rather than rehashing old platitudes, focussed and intelligent rather than effusive and contradictory, and emphasizing the personal labor needed for personal growth rather than claiming that enlightenment can occur without work and effort…the term "spiritual" describes awareness of a broader life meaning and/or domain that transcends the immediacy of everyday encounter and expediency.

The Changing Faces of Disease and Psycho-Spiritual Healing

While the majority of world cultures still remain in touch with shamans and spiritual dimensions, so-called "modern" people overlook the spiritual dimensions and encounters that permeate, coincide with, and are part and parcel of "encounter and expediency." For example, making a cup of tea, greeting relatives after an absence, or recovering from disease may be considered secular, "everyday" experiences. Yet many cultures imbue making a cup of tea, greeting relatives, or recovering from disease with deep spiritual significance. Sometimes this spiritual meaning is infused by the ceremony and ritual that pervades the behavior, creating a sense of sacred time and space. Sometimes it is found spontaneously, by the intuition of meaning behind a synchronistic coincidence, or by the insights of a third party like a counselor or shaman. The important thing is that such discovery of meaning often presages physical effects as well.

Recently, however, well-educated people in many European countries are getting back in touch with their healing traditions, seeking out traditional or paranormal healers (Kirfel, Lerner). Chinese and Japanese are reconsidering and renovating traditional paradigms of energy medicine, exercise, and native healing that had fallen into disuse after their adoption of Western medicine for its effectiveness on the battlefields of the 20th century (Kleinman, Lee). Despite many outward signs of "secularization" in America, when it comes to facing diseases and crises, a majority of patients turn their thoughts to religion, and wish their doctors would consider spiritual and religious issues with them. 77 percent say physicians should consider patients' spiritual needs; and half wish their physicians would pray with them! However, 68 percent said their physician had never discussed religious beliefs with them (King & Bushwick). The therapist-patient relationships is every bit as critical to healing in modern America as in Bali or Siberia.

Medical practice has long recognized the "placebo" effect: that a percentage of patients will recover from illnesses when an authoritative doctor they trust prescribes a medicine containing no active ingredients. The placebo effect has long been used in the clinical testing of new drugs: some of the patients are given the new drug, and others a placebo. If the recovery rate of the new drug is not significantly better than the placebo (which has no side-effects), then the drug is rarely approved. This mentality views the placebo as "worthless"; and therefore such new drugs are "little better than worthless." A more recent view asks instead, "if we can heal a certain percentage of patients using an inexpensive placebo with no side effects, how can this healing process be enhanced and utilized more broadly?!" A wide range of psychoneuro-immunological [PNI] research is beginning to demonstrate that patients' attitudes, particularly their faith in their physician and belief in their inherent wellness, indeed significantly affect their recovery rates.

Anthropologists from Skeat and Malinowski to Krippner have long reported the effects of spiritual connectedness in blocking pain. Firewalkers tread on thousand-degree coals; voodoo dancers eat glass and razor blades; Indians skewer their bodies; Pentecostal snake-handlers get themselves bitten by rattlesnakes; Brazilian Spiritualist surgeons cut open their patients without analgesics or anesthetics. In all of these cases, religious practitioners claim to feel no pain. Some of this may be explained in terms of hypnosis or by the burgeoning research in psychoneuro-immunology [although the mechanisms of hypnosis are not yet understood]. But the more remarkable fact is that in *some* such cases, the practitioners bodies retain no evidence of having been burned, punctured, poisoned, or sundered.

The physical mechanisms for these apparent miracles are as yet completely unknown, but such phenomena have tremendous implications for the future of medicine and health care. Just as some physicians who used to discount placebos are now eagerly utilizing the placebo effect to enhance their healing practices, so some doctors who used to dismiss psychic healing as charlatanry have moved to conceding the inherent value of studying the phenomena of religious healing.

In the above survey we have noted that religious views of disease pose opportunities for personal spiritual growth and psychosocial integration, as well as for genuine pain relief and healing. Next let us focus on some studies that may account for some of these phenomena.

Characteristics of the Healer

For several centuries now, doctors have witnessed Mesmer, Janet, Freud, Prince, and Sidis curing bodily ailments through psychological techniques (Bruce, 1910) casting doubt on traditional distinctions between physical and psychological (or somatic vs. mental) ailments. That a disease has mental rather than purely physical causes does not make it less painful, nor is a healing less significant if it reduces pain or symptoms by dealing with the mental aspects of the problem rather than by medicine or surgery.

Such examples lead some scholars to propose that the mechanism of religious healing is a kind of hypnotism or mental suggestion from the healer to the patient. The ambience, beliefs, and practices of Brazilian spiritualistic healing groups' combine to induce semi-hypnotic states and subsequent reactions that are acclaimed as cures (Quevedo, 1973a). British healer Eric Cuddon, whose pain relief through laying on of hands has been widely documented, believes that suggestion is a major factor at work in his own healing, although he agrees that suggestion alone cannot provide the whole explanation (Cuddon, 1968).

In another case, a doctor who had diagnosed three German women as having fatal diseases unsuccessfully collaborated with a faith healer. However, when the doctor told the women that they would be cured by a faith healer, all three patients recovered, although the faith healer had not been informed of the doctor's cooperation. The suggestion of the doctor, recognized as a symbol of authority, here seems to be as important as the suggestion of the healer himself (Belanger & del Vecchio, 1982).

Authoritatively Conveying an Image of the Disease and its Meaning

Shamanistic and psychotherapeutic healers maintain "metaphysical" views of the nature and origin of the diseases which they plan to heal, and communicating these views to their patients is important to the success of their healing (Beck, 1967). In Quebec, for example, Brunel found that Quebecois faith healers effectively use powerful battle imagery which appeals to their struggling patient (Belanger & Vecchio, 1982). Another common feature is the identifying of metaphoric significance to the body and its health. In religions as diverse as Tenrikyo, Christian Science, and Catholic Pentecostal healing, for example, difficulty in seeing, hearing, or swallowing might be diagnosed as an unwillingness to be receptive; headaches, as the improper use of the mind, and so on (McGuire, 1982; Becker, 1990).

Close Human Relationship between Patient and Healer

In order for the healer to convince the patient of a new view of the problem, patient and healer must share a close psychological rapport too often lacking in modern clinical medicine (Franks). Doctor Guarino, for example, holds that patients with weak constitutions are particularly susceptible to the beneficial effects suggested by healers with strong personalities. The healer awakens their "mechanisms of correlation," producing organic and systemic changes based on consolation, comprehension, and hope, of which medical physicians provide very limited amounts (Guarino, 1967). Compared to "the Western exorcism we call psychoanalysis," Halverson (1971) holds that (1) the patient-therapist relationship, (2) the social confidence in the efficacy of the rite, and (3) the interpretation that the patient is not personally responsible for his malady, are important factors in the more highly effective Sinhalese exorcism.

Characteristics of the Patient Conducive to Healing

In the 1950s, the Freiburg Institute studied 650 patients of Dr. Kurt Trampler, a mental healer in Germany (Strauch, 1963). Patients were given both psychological and physical tests to determine the changes in both their minds and bodies. The majority of patients were suffering from chronic illnesses that traditional medical care had failed to cure. Over a 14 month period of observation, 11 percent of the patients showed objective and permanent improvements, and an additional 50 percent reported that they "felt better" (subjectively), although objective measurements showed no difference in their medical conditions. In no case was the treatment found harmful.

Psychological testing of these 650 patients found those who were favorably predisposed to mental healing had subjectively better experiences than those who were not. This "positive" group tended to be less critical, but *less* imaginative, and *less* impressionable than the "skeptical" group. The group who felt that they had had positive improvements tended to be rural or working-class middle-aged women, whereas the "skeptical" group tended to be younger educated urban males (Strauch, 1963). This Freiburg study is significant in showing the role of expectation in the "effectiveness" of healing, but it also raises doubts about "hypnotic" theories.

Psychic healers are often enshrouded by sensationalistic rumors of miraculous healings promulgated by a word-of-mouth grapevine network. One study of Brazilian healer Ze Arigo (Jose Pedro de Freitas) attempted to contact 836 of his clients. Of those, 25 percent could not be analyzed, 50 percent felt no significant change, and only 15.5 percent felt improved. The investigator concluded that propaganda, hypnosis, and hysteria were responsible for the successes of Arigo (Quevedo, 1973b). However, the fact that many of these healings were "subjective" need not detract from their value. After all, most patients desire to *feel* better, rather than to feel the same but to be told that their conditions are measurably improved.

The Role of Intense Faith and Hope

Bender's research on intense emotional tensions in healers, stemming from feelings of sympathy, desire to help, and related factors, led him to hypothesize that these tensions build up "a charged field," that causes patients to accept the healer's suggestions and be cured. He cites several examples of people cured by Jung and Rehder which fit this model (Bender, 1964). However, these examples focus more and more on the patient or victim himself, rather than on the healer or healer-patient relationship.

For healers who do not practice physical contact, the faith of the patients themselves is surely a very important variable. Consider the situation in which a patient goes either to a sacred location (such as Lourdes, Ste. Anne de Baupré, or Tenri), or to a charismatic religious healer (such as Justa Smith) seeking healing (Chesanow, 1979). Such healing situations are more difficult to place in "control groups," but a number of studies have been conducted which give us some insight into the nature of this healing process. This principle is most clearly at work in cases like those of the healings at Lourdes and similar shrines, which have been carefully verified over a long period of time, but which do not depend on the touch, suggestion, or relation of any single personal healer (Leuret & Meng, 1957).

Immunity and Pain Desensitization Through Ecstatic States

Recent studies in the neurosciences show that intense emotional states create biochemicals which dull pain and can evoke ecstatic states. In Latin America, *vidente* healing uses such ecstatic and intense emotions to facilitate healing (DeRios, 1984). Similarly, members of the Free Pentecostal Holiness Church have handled very hot flames, been bitten by serpents, and ingested poisonous doses of strychnine, without any harmful effects. Study of these paranormal abilities of people in ecstatic trance may harbor great practical value to the medical community (Schwartz, 1960).

We have just noted a number of elements which lead to the successes of faith healers, traditional healers, or paranormal healers: factors including their hypnotic, suggestive, or persuasive views and personalities, the close relationships between the healers and the patients, the faith of the patients in their practitioners, and the strong emotional elements of expectation and even ecstasy as factors.

Characteristics of the Brains of Mental Healers

The above studies have recognized that not only the physical placement of a healer's hands or body, but the attitude and mental state of the healer is critical to the success of mental healing. Some "bio-engineers" from the Soviet Union have directed what they call "bio-radiant" energy from the brains of the healers to treated subjects (Mirahorian, 1967). Many religions which practice mental healing have also acknowledged this factor. ESP tests carried out with French healer Aldo Moreau de la Mense seemed to demonstrate a high level of general ESP ability, but no precognitive abilities (Onetto, 1976). Other scholars have identified psychological and physiological similarities between meditation and the therapeutic touch; a state of mind in the healer similar to a state of meditation seems to be necessary for healing to occur (Borelli, 1981).

Experienced healers like Enrico Tomasetti occasionally find that their hands respond to the sick patient's condition, independent of the healer's volition or intention. In other words, if the healer is sensitive to the patient's conditions, "The performer does not intervene rationally, but must be capable of reacting with his own muscular system to the least variations in the field of forces connected with the environment and particularly with the patient."(Borello, 1967: 91). Chinese and Japanese studies of *ki* (*qi*) indicate that one or more inadequately understood para-physical energies connect the nerves and meridian system, not only in acupuncture and acupressure, but at a distance through mental activity (cf. Lee, Motoyama, 1986: 60 ff.). However, the findings to date suggest some empirical evidence for the medical validity of the therapeutic touch; it seems specifically indicated in a range of acute and chronic illnesses, and is "an extremely safe adjunctive (medical) modality"(Proudfoot, 1981).

Prayer and Absent Religious Healing

In addition to healings which may be explained by models of "psychosomatic" faith healing or of "laying on of hands," a third area of healing deserving study includes cases where the work of the healer is unknown to the patient. One classical example is that of Jesus and the centurion, wherein the patient neither saw nor knew the healer (Matthew 8). In this case, the centurion [a third party] asked the healer [Jesus] to heal his servant a long distance away, and the servant was discovered to have recovered at the same time that the healing was requested. To be sure, in this instance, Jesus praised the faith of the centurion, but neither the centurion nor Jesus were present with the sick servant, nor did the sick servant have any way of knowing the hour at which Jesus agreed to heal him. Only the temporal coincidence of the healing seems to indicate a connection between their dialogue and the patient's improvement. In such cases, neither physical contact nor the faith of the patient seems sufficient to explain the "miracle" involved.

Like pre-modern physics, medical science rejects influence at a distance [the claim that healing can be effected from afar, as in intercessory prayer]. Physicians prefer to regard such events as coincidence, in spite of the fact that communication without known physical means of transmission has been proven possible according to exacting scientific standards (Booth, 1957). Often classified as "absent healing," examples of sudden recovery where no material nor psychical mechanisms other than the prayer of a distant person can apparently account for the healing have been catalogued through the ages (Hebda, 1975). William Braud's research suggests that visualization and imagery techniques can effect the quality of one's own blood *even after it has been removed from the body and put in a test tube in another room.* If further research bears out Broad's findings, how much more probable is it that blood still coursing through human veins and brains will be influenced by our mental states, as indeed Carl Simonton proposes in his imagery treatments for cancer.

In 1997, Targ, Schlitz, Braud, and others gathered an impressive array of evidence that in fact intercessory prayer can have effects on healing—even at a distance, and even when the praying was unknown or timing unconfirmed by the "recipient" patient. Then the *Annals of Internal Medicine* rocked the medical world with Astin and Harkness' systematic review of randomized trials—which essentially validated what Targ, Broad, Dossey, and others had been saying—but in a far more famous professional forum. Some reports of "failures" in prayer do not invalidate what other patients feel to be their "successes." In addition to measuring the physical improvement of each patient's condition, there is also a need for further evaluation of the psycho-social benefits (or damage) incurred by patients who turn to prayer to supplement their medical care.

Instances where the patient is an infant or delirious (and therefore has no consciousness of the activity of the healer), and the healer does not physically touch the patient, also provide strong evidence that neither the touch nor the faith of the patient alone are sufficient to explain religious healing (Puxley, 1966). Examples of this sort can be found in many healing religions today, but not until more examples are gathered and analyzed can their common elements and distinctive features be adequately understood (e.g. Peel, 1987). In the meantime, we might recognize the possibility that behind these phenomena are forces at work which are not yet adequately studied or researched by the medical and psychological sciences.

There is yet much room for fruitful gathering and interpretation of data in this area by social scientists and scholars of religions, as well as by medical and psychiatric professionals. Doctors have long relied on drugs whose probable effects were well known, without knowing the precise mechanisms of those drugs within the brain or body. Similarly, hypnotists have long deadened pain and cured bad habits and personality disorders, without knowing the "mechanisms" by which hypnotism works. The above literature and experiments document that a more holistic view of the healing process—including the patients' physical environment, psychological state, and belief system—might indeed be conducive to improvement of the physical and/or mental health of medical patients. Whatever the mechanisms involved, if it is possible to improve health through such means, we should work in that direction. Taking all due precaution against fraud and quackery, we may also gain a fuller understanding of the human potential and the workings of the human mind and body.

This chapter—and indeed this book—is only an introduction to some of the problems and prospects for alternative methods of healing. The physicians and contributors to this volume recognize the importance of mental as well as physical, or better, of holistic and comprehensive as well as analytic and microscopic, approaches to health and healing. The appended Bibliography gives interested readers resources for further research.

Bibliography

Aakster, C. W. (1986). "Concepts in alternative medicine." *Social Science and Medicine*, 22 (2), 265-273.

Astin, J. A., Harknes, E., Ernst, E. (2000). "The efficacy of 'distant healing': a systematic review of randomized trials." *Annals of Internal Medicine*, June 6, 2000, 132 (11), 903-10.

Bahr, D. M., Gregorio, J., Lopez, D. I., & Alvarez, A. *Piman Shamanism and Staying Sickness*. Tucson: University of Arizona, 1974.

Bartlett, Laile. (1978) "Bernard Grad and energy." *Human Behavior*, 7 (6), 28-32.

Beck, Robert. (1967). "Some proto-therapeutic elements in the practice of the shaman," *History of Religions.* 6, 303-327.

Becker, Carl. (1990). "Religious healing in 19th century 'New Religions,'" *Religion.* 20, 199-215.

―――(1991). "From pain to philosophy: Functions of art and religion." *Journal of Religion and Psychical Research.* 14 (3), 144-153

―――(1992.) "Indian, Japanese, and psychoanalytic research on meditation" *Tsukuba Chiiki Kenkyu.* 10 (3), 121-130.

―――(1996). "Effects of human values on scientific objectivity," *In Depth--Journal for Values and Public Policy.* 5 (1), 89-112.

Belanger, Louis, & del Vecchio, Lucia. (1982). "The art of Quebecois healers: a cultural good repudiated by the dominant class," *Le Bulletin PSILOG.* 1, 9-16.

Bender, Hans. (1964). "Miraculous healings in the affective field," *Zeitschrift fur Parapsychologie und Grenzgebeite fur Psychologie.* 7(1), 4-24.

Booth, Gotthard. (1957). "Science and spiritual healing," *Proceedings of Four Conferences of Parapsychological Studies.* New York: Parapsychological Foundation, pp. 53-55.

Borelli, M. D. (1981). "Meditation and Therapeutic Touch," Heidt & Borelli, pp. 40-46.

Borello, Erminia de Stefano. (1967). "Education to improve recognition of the work of healers," *Metapsichica Rivista Italiana di Parapsicologia.* 22, 89-101.

Braud, William G. (1990). "Distant mental influence of rate of hemolysis of human red blood cells." *Journal of the American Society for Psychical Research*, 84 (1), 1-24.

Bruce, Addington. (1910). "Remarkable cures effected by four great experts without the aid of drugs or surgeons' tools," *American Magazine.* 71, 71-80.

Cadoret, Remi & Paul, G. I. (1961). "An unorthodox method of treatment on wound healing in mice," *International Journal of Parapsychology.* 3 (2), 5-24.

Chesanow, Neil. (1979). "Is it time to take psychic healing seriously?" *Family Health.* 11, pp. 22 ff.

Cuddon, Eric. (1968). "The relief of pain by the laying on of hands. Suggestion? Restoration of electro-static balance? Emanation? Illusion?" *International Journal of Parapsychology.* 10 (1), 85-92.

Dean, Douglas. (1983). *An Examination of Infra-red and Ultra-Violet Techniques to Test for Changes in Water Following the Laying-on of Hands.* Saybrook Institute: Ph.D. Dissertation.

Dein, Simon. (1992). "The management of illness by a Filipino psychic surgeon: A Western physician's impression." *Social Science and Medicine,* 34 (4), 461-464.

DeRios, Marlene Dobkin. (1984). "The Vidente phenomenon in third world traditional healing: an Amazonian example," *Medical Anthropology,* 6, 60-70.

Dossey, Larry. (1996). *Prayer is Good Medicine: How to Reap the Healing Benefits of Prayer.* San Francisco: Harper San Francisco.

——(1999). *Reinventing Medicine: Beyond Mind-Body to a New Era of Healing.* San Francisco: Harper San Francisco.

Edge, Hoyt L. (1993). "The medium as healer and clown: An interpretation of Balinese mediumship." *Journal of the American Society for Psychical Research,* 87(2), 171-183.

Elgium, Gina H. (1967). "Psychokinesis in Experimental Tumerogenesis," *Zeitschrift fur Parapsychologie und Grenzgebeite der Psychologie.* 110, 4-60.

Eliade, M. (1964). *Shamanism: Archaic Techniques of Ecstasy.* Princeton, NJ: Princeton Univ. Press.

Fahler, J. & Keil, H. H. J. (1976). "Nina Kulagina: a strong case for PK involving directly observable movements of objects," *European Journal of Parapsychology.* 1 (2), 36-44.

Frank, J.D. & J. B. (1991). *Persuasion and healing: A Comparative Study of Psychotherapy.* (3rd ed., sponsored by NIMH). Baltimore, MD: Johns Hopkins University Press.

Fuller, Robert. (1987). "Unorthodox medicine and American religious life," *The Journal of Religion.* 50-65.

Grad, Bernard. (1963, 1964). "A telekinetic effect on plant growth," *International Journal of Parapsychology.* 5 (2), 117-133; 6 (4), 473-498.

Guarino, Alberto. (1967). "A medical view of healers," *Rivista Italiana di Parapsicologia* 22: 1-8.

Halverson, John. (1971). "Dynamics of exorcism," *History of Religions.* 10 (4), 334-359.

Hearne, Keith M. T. 1982. "'Energy Flow' between healer and patient?" *Journal of the Society for Psychical Research.* 51 (792), 382-384.

Hebda, Hillard. (1975). *An Inquiry into Unorthodox Healing.* Governor's State University, Illinois: M.A. Thesis.

Heidt, P. & Borelli, M. D. (eds.) (1981). *Therapeutic Touch: A Book of Readings.* New York: Springer.

Hermanns, Matthias. (1970). *Schamanen, Pseudoschamanen, Erlöser und Heilbringer.* Weisbaden, Germany: F. Steiner.

King, D. E. & Bushwick, B. (1994). "Beliefs and attitudes of hospital inpatients about faith healing and prayer." *Journal of Family Practice,* 39 (4), 349-352.

Kirfel, Bernhard. (1984). "Heilkundige in der Eifel [Medical Science in the Eifel]." *Curare,* 7 (4), 239-258.

Kleinman, Arthur, & Sung, L. H. (1979). "Why do indigenous practitioners successfully heal?" *Social Science and Medicine,* 13B (1), 7-26.

Krieger, Dolores. (1975). "Therapeutic Touch: the imprimatur of nursing," *American Journal of Nursing.* 75 (5), 784-787.

Lee, Yuehting, & Hu, Pei Cheng. (1993). "The effect of Chinese Qi gong exercises and therapy on diseases and health." *Journal of Indian Psychology,* 11 (1-2), 9-18.

Lerner, Michael. (1994). *Choices in Healing: Integrating the Best of Conventional and Complementary Approaches to Cancer.* Cambridge, MA: MIT Press.

Leuret, Francois & Meng, Heinrich. (1957). "Implications of the 'Miracles of Lourdes'," *Proceedings of Four Conferences of Parapsychological Studies.* New York: Parapsychological Foundation, pp. 80-84.

Marinho, Jarbas. (1976). "Kirlian photography and evidence of energy transmission from one person to another," *Psi Comunicación.* 2, 65-69.

McGuire, Meredith. (1982). "Healing: Conformity, Community, Order, Power," in *Pentecostal Catholics.* Philadelphia: Temple U. Press, pp. 163-183.

Mirahorian, Levon. (1967). "Parapsychotherapy in medical pathology," *Metapsichica Rivista Italiana di Parapsicologia.* 22, 79-88.

Motoyama, Hiroshi. (1986). *Psi to Ki no Kankei [The Relation of Psi to Ki Energy].* Tokyo: Shukyou Shinrigaku Kenkyusho.

Onetto, Brenio. (1976). "Latin American Healers," *Psi Communicación.* 2, 33-40.

Peel, Robert. (1987). *Spiritual Healing in a Scientific Age.* NewYork: Harper &Row.

Pelletier, Kenneth. (1979). *Holistic Medicine.* New York: Delacorte Press.

Proudfoot, Martin. (1981). "Scientific medicine and therapeutic touch," Heidt & Borelli, pp. 98-106.

Puxley, H. L. (1966). "Opening Address" to Parapsychology Foundation Conference on Religion and Parapsychology, in *International Journal of Parapsychology.* 8 (2), 290-294.

Quevedo, Oscar. (1973). "The Problem of healing, Part I," *Revista de Parapsicologia.* I (3), 4-11, I (4), 4-13.

Schlitz M, & Braud W. (1997). "Distant intentionality and healing: assessing the evidence." *Alternative Therapies in Health and Medicine.* Nov, 3(6), 62-73.

Schwartz, Berthold. (1960). "Ordeal by serpents, fire, and strychnine," *Psychiatric Quarterly.* 34, 405-429.

Sicher F., & Targ E., Moore D. 2nd, Smith H. S. (1998). "A randomized double-blind study of the effect of distant healing in a population with advanced AIDS. Report of a small scale study." *West Journal of Med.* Dec, 169 (6), 356-63.

Simonton, O. C. (1978). *Getting Well Again.* Los Angeles: J. P. Tarcher.

Strauch, Inge. (1963). "Medical aspects of 'mental healing,'" *International Journal of Parapsychology.* 5 (2), 135-165.

Targ, E. (1997). "Evaluating distant healing: a research review." *Alternative Therapies in Health and Medicine.* 3 (6), 74-8.

Walsh, Roger N. (1990). *The Spirit of Shamanism.* Los Angeles, CA: Jeremy P. Tarcher.

Worrall, Ambrose & Olga. (1968). *The Miracle Healers.* New York: Signet Books.